CROCHET
FOR
ABSOLUTE BEGINNERS

LUISA DE SANTI
CRAFTERIE PRESS

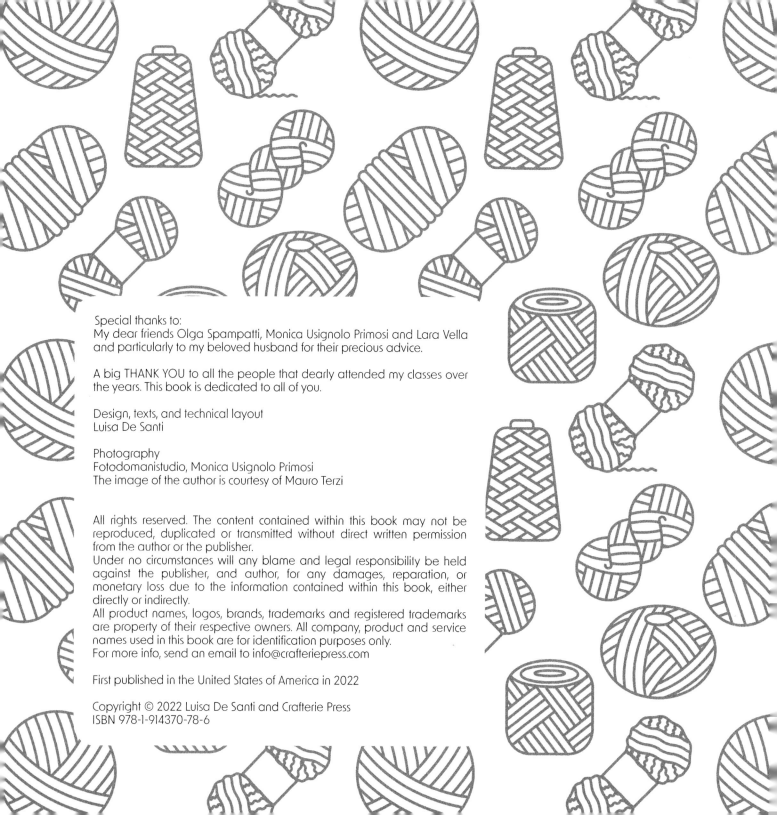

Special thanks to:
My dear friends Olga Spampatti, Monica Usignolo Primosi and Lara Vella and particularly to my beloved husband for their precious advice.

A big THANK YOU to all the people that dearly attended my classes over the years. This book is dedicated to all of you.

Design, texts, and technical layout
Luisa De Santi

Photography
Fotodomanistudio, Monica Usignolo Primosi
The image of the author is courtesy of Mauro Terzi

First published in the United States of America in 2022

Copyright © 2022 Luisa De Santi and Crafterie Press
ISBN 978-1-914370-78-6

CONTENTS

PATTERNS AND PROJECTS

SPECIAL AMIGURUMI PROJECT

ART INSPIRATIONAL BOX

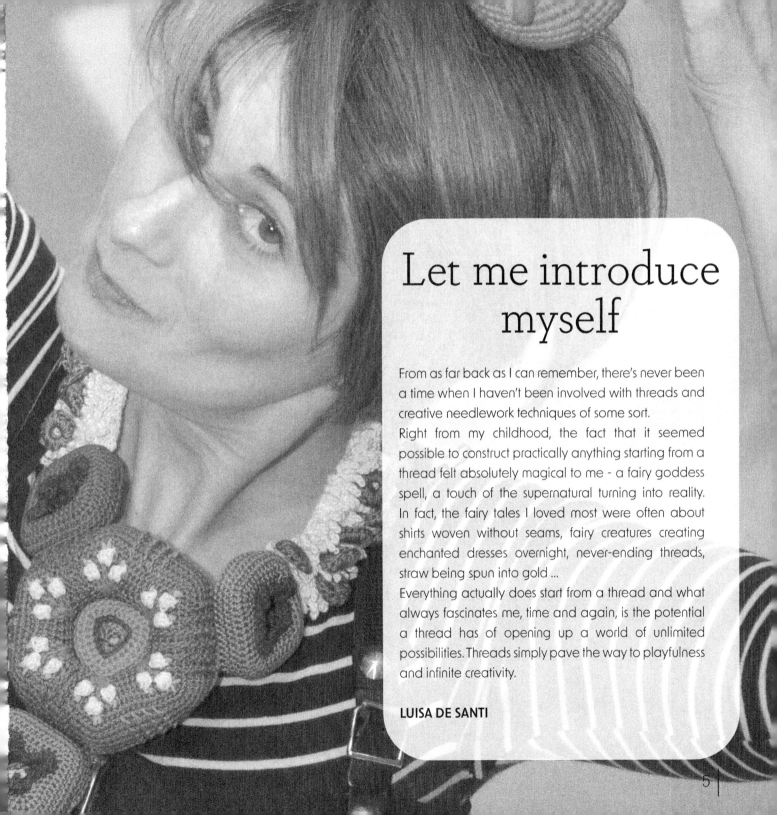

Let me introduce myself

From as far back as I can remember, there's never been a time when I haven't been involved with threads and creative needlework techniques of some sort.

Right from my childhood, the fact that it seemed possible to construct practically anything starting from a thread felt absolutely magical to me - a fairy goddess spell, a touch of the supernatural turning into reality. In fact, the fairy tales I loved most were often about shirts woven without seams, fairy creatures creating enchanted dresses overnight, never-ending threads, straw being spun into gold ...

Everything actually does start from a thread and what always fascinates me, time and again, is the potential a thread has of opening up a world of unlimited possibilities. Threads simply pave the way to playfulness and infinite creativity.

LUISA DE SANTI

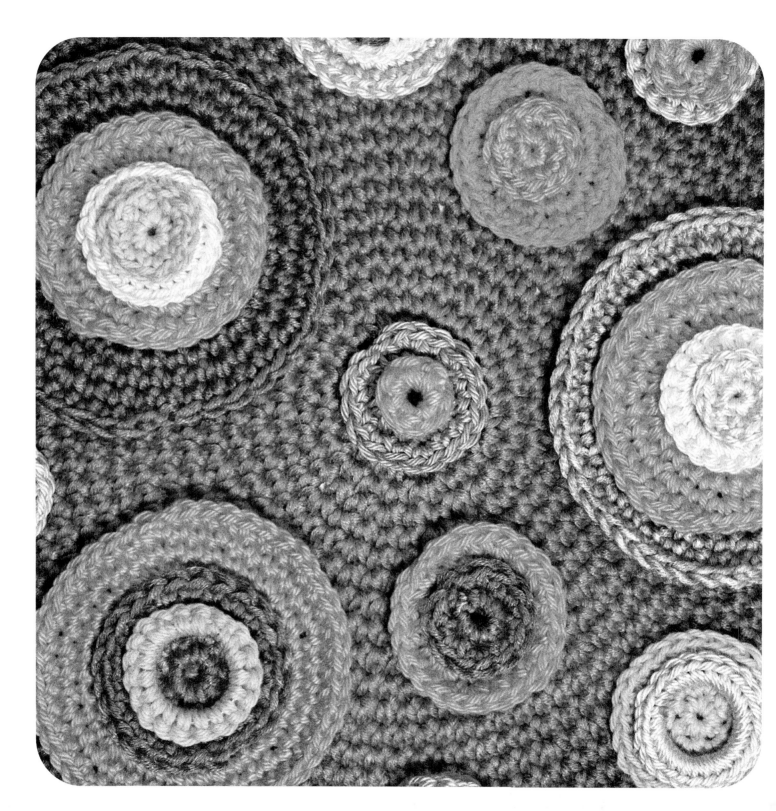

Magical Crochets

Do you feel you are totally out of your depth with a crochet hook and that you'll never learn to make really striking crochet pieces?

Well here's the good news... this book is for you!

You don't need to know a whole lot of stitches or resort to magical crochet spells: all you need to know is how to stitch the basics. When your foundation is solid, building from there is quite simple.

The secret is to learn to crochet smoothly, to mix and match your yarn colors and to follow simple instructions as you go along.

Are you ready to start your journey into creativity with me?

FINE THEN, LEAF OVER AND LET'S GET STARTED!

ACCESS LUISA DE SANTI CROCHET ACADEMY

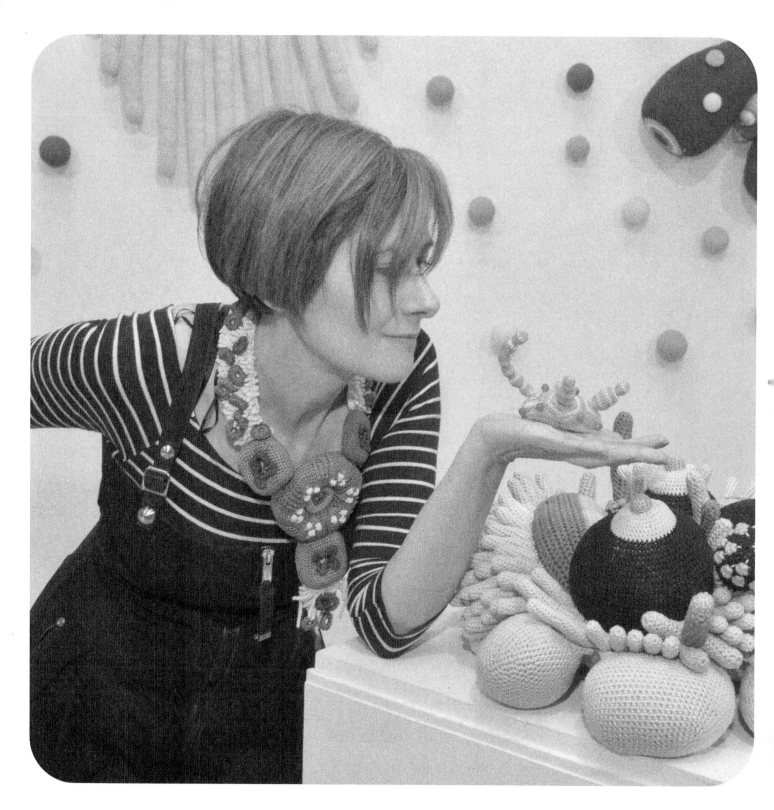

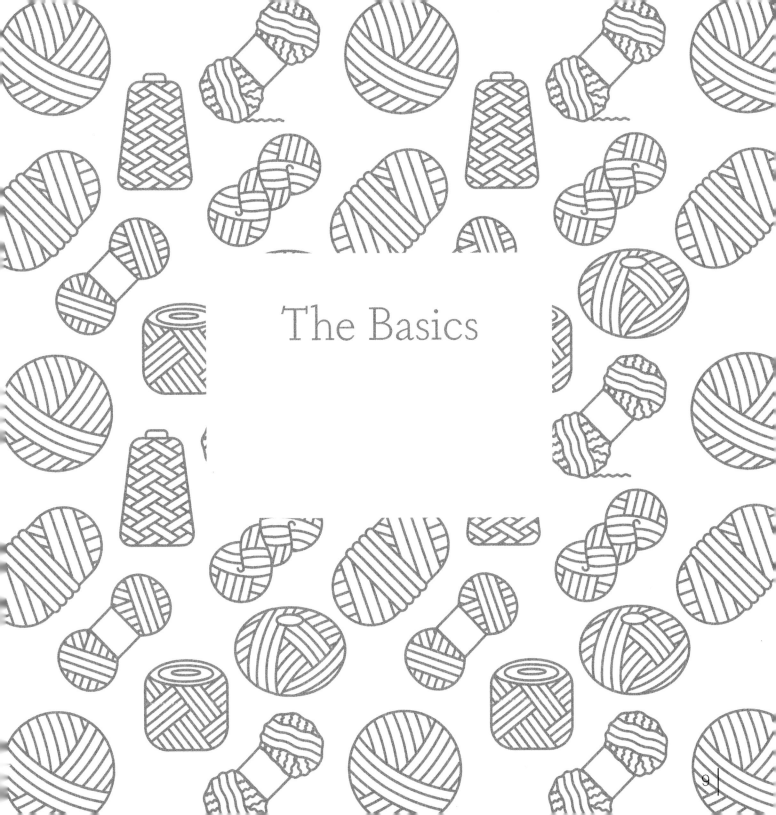

The Basics

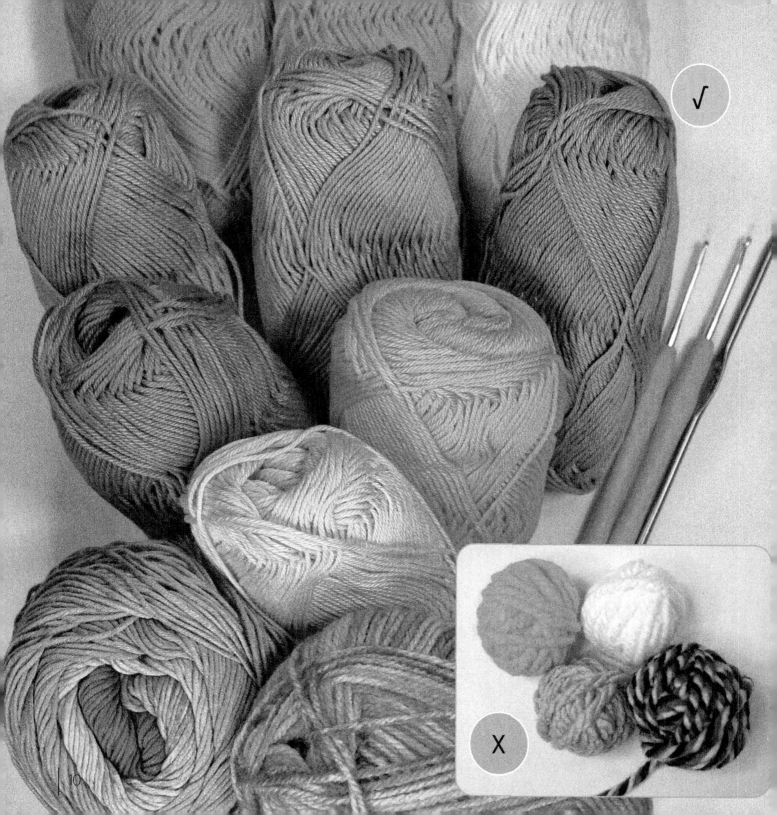

√

X

Yarns and Tools

YARNS

How do you choose the right yarn for your projects and skill level?

Each pattern in this book provides detailed and accurate yarn specifications. Keep in mind that thicker yarns are easier to work with: it's easier to identify stitches and rows, and where you need to insert your hook. Plus any errors or other irregularities in your work will pop out and become more evident. If you need to go out and purchase some yarn, carefully read the label on each skein and check the weight (in oz and g) and the total length (in yds and m) on each single skein, then cross-reference the data with the instructions I give you for each pattern. Although it might be of the same weight, a thicker yarn will be shorter in length.

beginner, first-time crochet project: Super Bulky (6)	1.75ozs=32.5yds (50g=30m),
	hook size N/P-15 (10mm)
beginner, second-time crochet project: Bulky (5)	1.75ozs=90yds (50g=82.5m)
	hook size J-10 (6mm)
beginner, third- time crochet project: Light (3)	1.75ozs=145yds (50g=133m),
	hook size G-6 (4 mm)

Refer to the chart above for further details and suggestions.

Check the label for care instructions, washing temperature (if washable) and whether it can be dry-cleaned or not. The best brands will specify all these details very clearly. If you buy small-scale production yarns, ask the seller to supply you with the above information.

When choosing the colors for your beginner projects, choose solid, light and bright-colored yarns. Avoid blacks, dark browns and colors that may be tiring to the eye. You can also use gradient yarns and radial-gradient (ombre) yarns, but do so after you have done some practice.

If you have any questions, don't be shy and feel free to write and ask me directly!

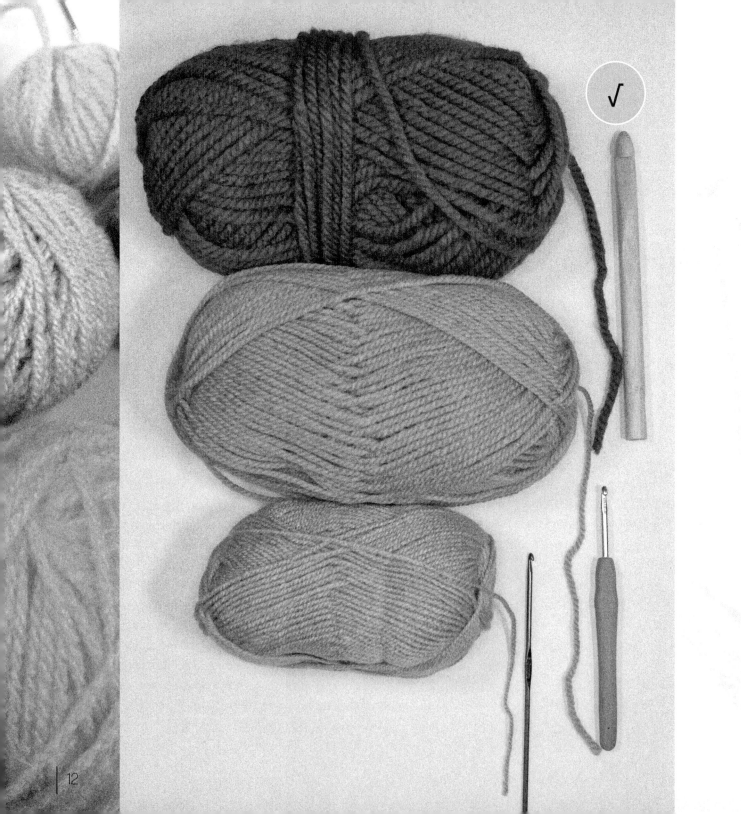

TOOLS

You will obviously need crochet hooks, but also yarn needles and stitch markers for your projects.

CROCHET HOOKS

There is a very large variety of crochet hooks available and they can either be in plastic, steel and/or wood. Usually the thicker crochet hooks (perfect for beginners) are in plastic or wood, while the thinner ones (for advanced crocheters) are made of steel.

Yarn labels will also always specify the best hook to use for that yarn. The hook size on the label can vary according to the brand and the origin of the yarn, and it can be in both letters and numbers, so I recommend that you always refer to the size expressed in millimeters. Sometimes the hook size is specified with a range of values (i.e. 3-4mm). In these cases, it's up to you to choose the hook size based on your own individual crocheting tension.

It helps to do a test swatch before starting on a new project. If you want your crochet fabric to turn out soft and cosy (perfect for wearable projects) choose a thicker sized hook, if you want your crochet fabric to be stiff and flexible at the same time (perfect for stuffed projects like amigurumi), choose a thinner one.

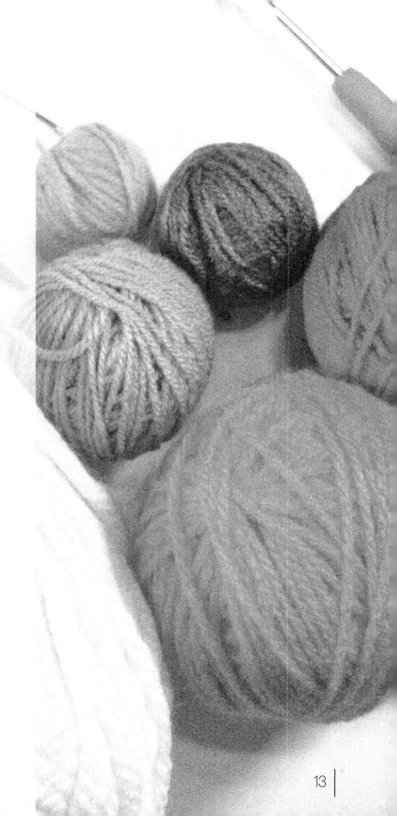

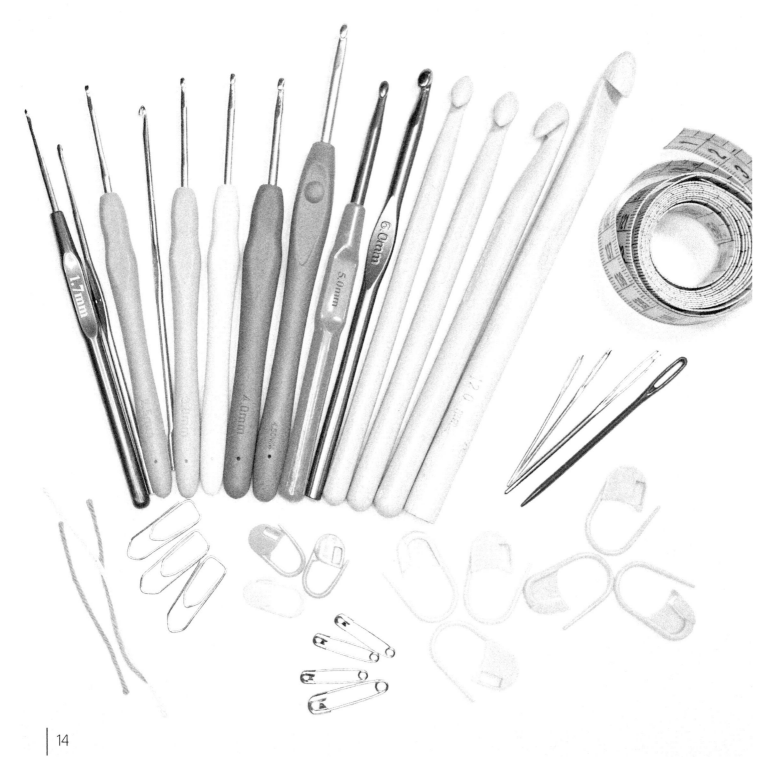

YARN NEEDLES

Both plastic needles (perfect for travelling) and steel needles (mostly nickel-plated or gold-plated) are available on the market. Needles differentiate in thickness, length, tip (round or sharp) and shape of the eye (round eye, medium or long eye). Every technique requires its own specific type of needle. No panic, relax! In this book, as for all beginner projects, we will use yarn needles that are very simple to identify: they have a rounded tip and a rather long, wide eye. The only thing to really check is the thickness of your yarn and that the yarn needle you select has a sufficiently large eye for the yarn you intend to use. Also check that the yarn needle has a rounded tip so that it will pass through crochet fabric without tearing or splitting the yarn fibers.

STITCH MARKERS

Stitch markers are small tools used to mark the first stitch in a round when crocheting continuous crochet circles. They are simply visual references that mark your progress and show you where the beginning of a round is located. If you don't have stitch markers you can get creative and replace them using safety pins, paper clips or simply a small length of scrap yarn instead.

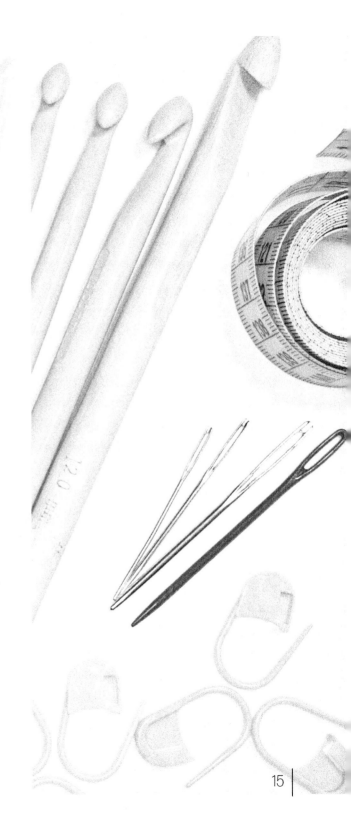

All about hooks

See the table below for hook size conversion data:

METRIC	US
2.25 mm	B-1
2.75 mm	C-2
3.125 mm	D-3
3.75 mm	F-5
4 mm	G-6
4.25	G
4.5 mm	7
5 mm	H-8
5.25	I
5.5 mm	I-9
5.75	J
6 mm	J-10
6.5 mm	K-10½
8 mm	L-11
9 mm	M/N-13
10 mm	N/P-15
11.5 mm	P-16
15 mm	P/Q

№	mm
14	0,50
12	0,60
10	0,75
8	0,90
6	1,00
4	1,25
2	1,50
0	1,75

№	mm		№	mm
2/0	2,0		10/0	6,0
3/0	2,3		7	7,0
4/0	2,5		8	8,0
5/0	3,0		10	10,0
6/0	2,5		12	12,0
70/0	4,0		15	15,0
7,5/0	4,5		20	20,0
8/0	5,0			
9/0	5,5			

How to chain stitch

Holding the yarn: step 1. Loop yarn around little finger and forefinger

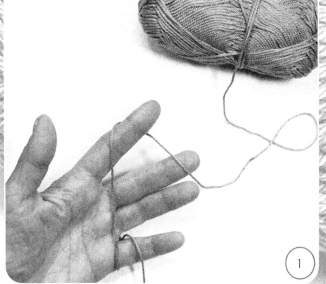

Holding the yarn: step 2. Hold back section of yarn firmly between thumb and forefinger

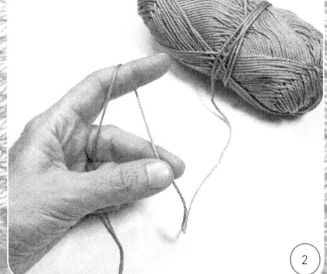

LET ME SHOW YOU

How to hold the hook - how to insert the hook

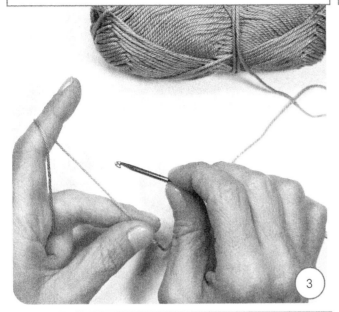

- slip hook under yarn from back to front

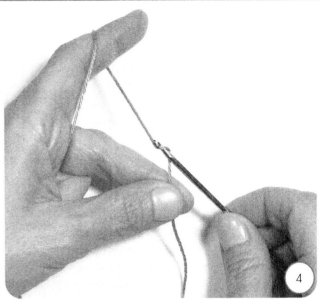

- rotate hook clockwise once to twist yarn

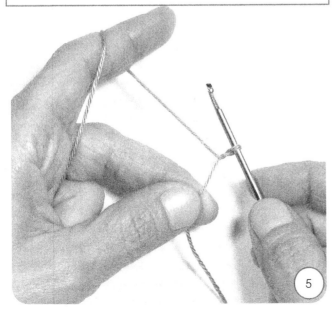

- rest hook and yarn twist loop on middle finger

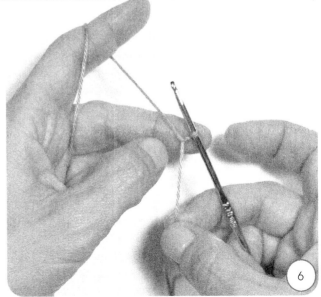

Chain stitch: step 4. Pressing yarn twist loop and tail firmly between thumb and forefinger, slip hook under yarn and wrap yarn over from back to front (2 loops on hook)

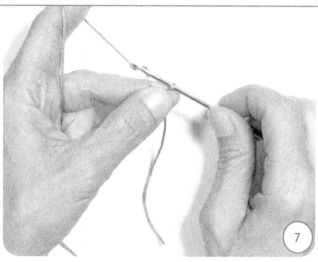

7

Chain stitch step 5. Pull on hook to draw second loop through first loop. Repeat steps 4 and 5 as many times as required

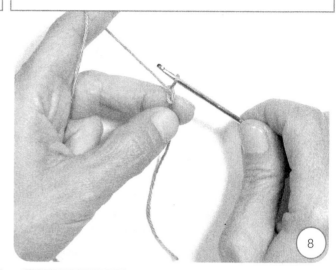

8

Here is a foundation chain made of 10 chains (counting chains from 1 to 10)

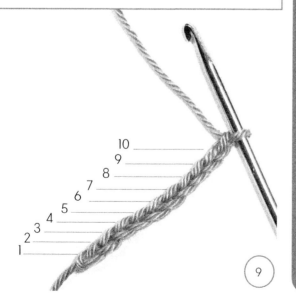

9

How to slip stitch

Step 1: insert the hook into a chain (or a stitch) and wrap the yarn over the hook

Step 2: pull through to draw up a loop (2 loops on hook)

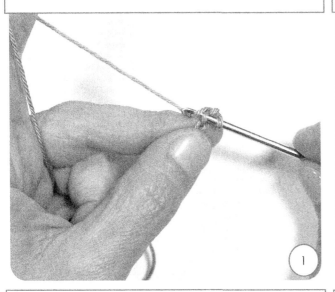

Step 3: draw the second loop through the first loop in one motion: you have completed your first slip stitch

to make more slip stitches, repeat steps 1 to 3.

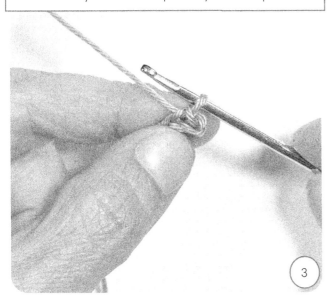

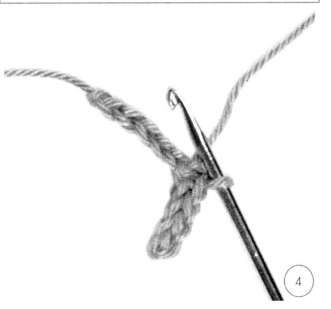

How to single crochet

Step 1: insert the hook into a chain (or a stitch) then wrap the yarn over the hook

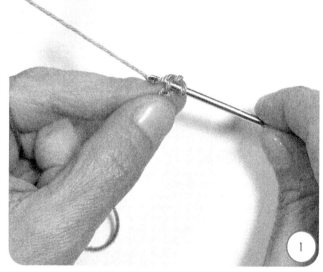

Step 2: pull through to draw up a loop (2 loops on your hook)

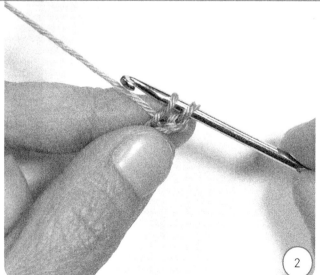

Step 3: wrap the yarn over your hook again and draw it through both the loops on your hook in one motion

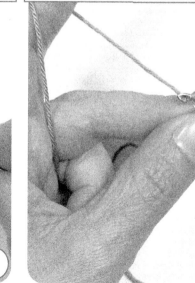

Your first single crochet is complete

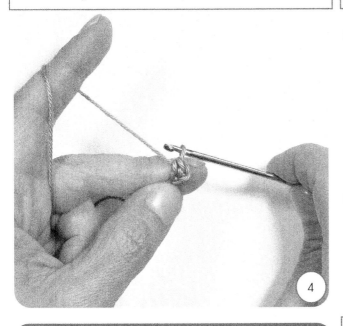

to make more single crochets, repeat steps 1 to 3.

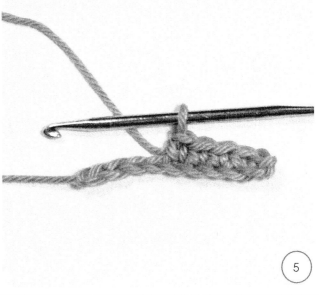

How to make a chain ring

Make a number of chains then insert your hook into the first chain

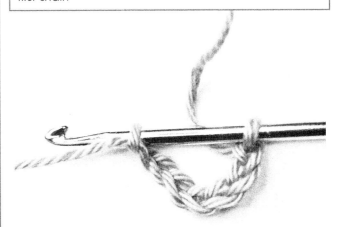

Wrap the yarn over the hook, then pull the yarn through both the chain and the loop on your hook in one motion (you have essentially made a slip stitch to close the ring)

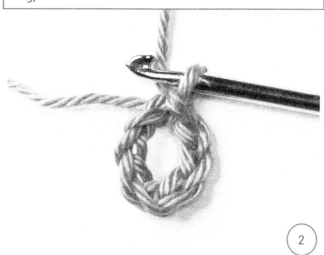

(2)

ROUND 1: single crochet as instructed in pattern

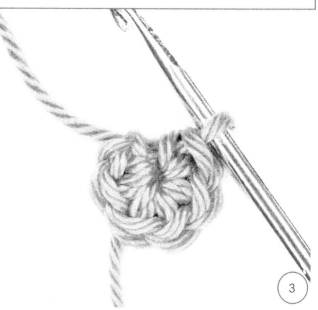

(3)

Insert the hook into the first stitch of the round

(4)

Make the first single crochet of the second round

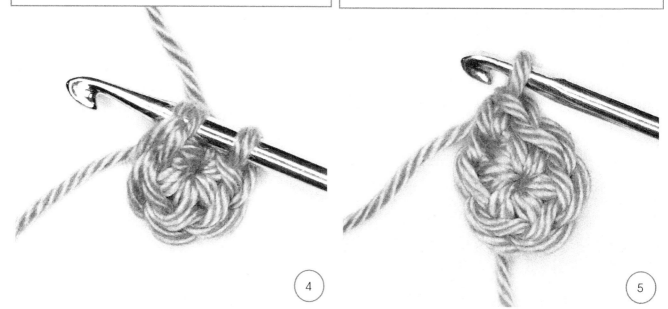

(5)

Mark this first single crochet with a stitch marker

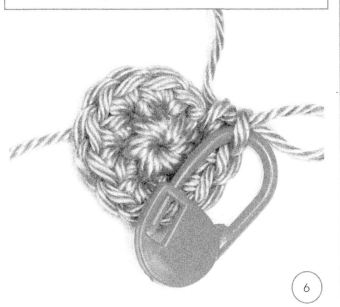

(6)

How to cut yarn and fasten off

When you reach the end of your pattern instructions, make 1 slip stitch, then cut the yarn leaving a tail about 10 inches long. Insert the tail end through the last loop left on the hook, remove the hook and pull on the tail to close the loop. Thread the yarn tail into a yarn needle

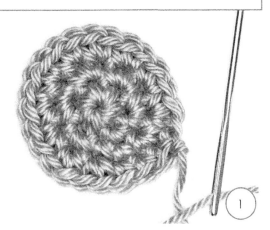

(1)

Fasten off by working the yarn tail into the back of your work

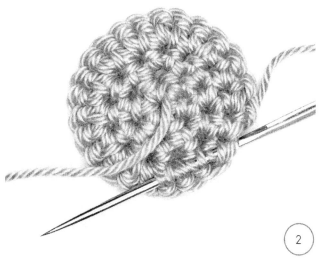

(2)

How to identify the right and wrong sides of your fabric

The side of the stitch that faces you while crocheting is the right side (front, or front surface) of your fabric. The side of the stitch that doesn't face you while crocheting is the wrong side (back, or back surface) of your fabric. They aren't actually "right" or "wrong", you only need to know how to identify them: front surface (right), back surface (left)

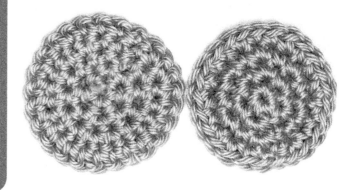

More ways of inserting the hook into a foundation chain

1. You can insert your hook into both the top loop and the back bar of the chain

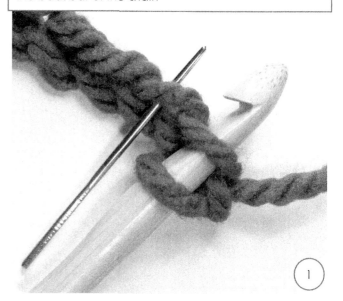

2. You can insert your hook into both the top and the bottom loops of the chain

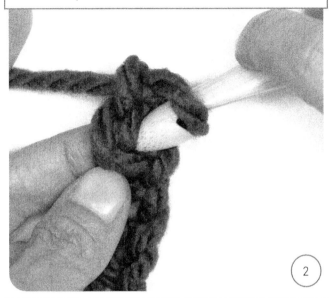

(2)

3. You can insert your hook only into the back bar of the chain

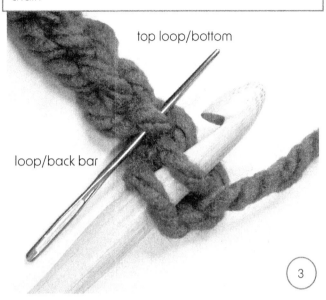

top loop/bottom

loop/back bar

(3)

the 3 ways of inserting a hook into a foundation chain

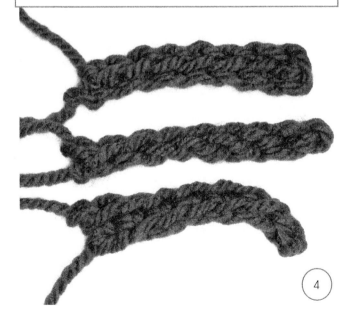

(4)

How to form a yarn loop

To form a yarn loop, wind yarn around forefinger holding yarn tail firmly between thumb and ring finger.

Insert hook under the yarn loop, yarn over and pull up a loop.

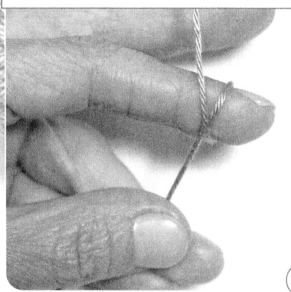

(1)

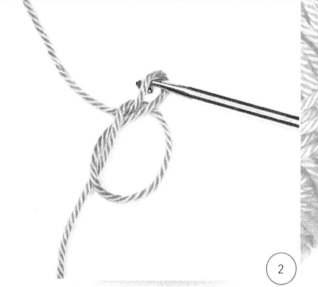

(2)

LET ME SHOW YOU

Chain 1, then make the number of stitches stated in pattern instructions.

Pull firmly on the tail yarn to close the starting loop and to pull the stitches in the first round together.

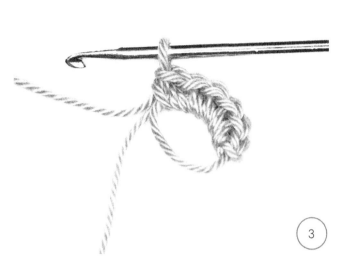

(3)

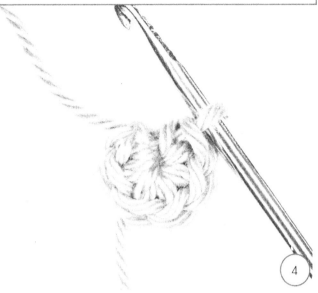

(4)

How to double crochet

Chain 3 (this group of chains replaces your first double crochet)

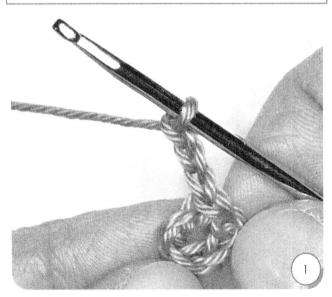

(1)

Wrap yarn over hook.

Insert the hook into the chain ring (or into a stitch), wrap yarn over hook and pull up a loop back through the chain ring (or stitch).

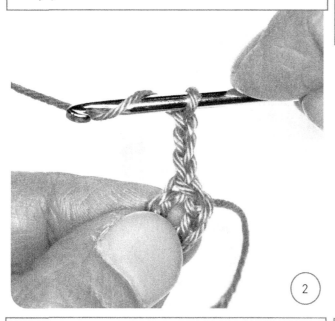

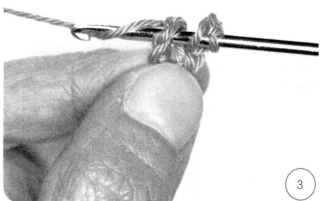

You now have 3 loops on hook. Yarn over and pull through 2 loops.

You now have 2 loops on hook. Yarn over and pull through the remaining 2 loops.

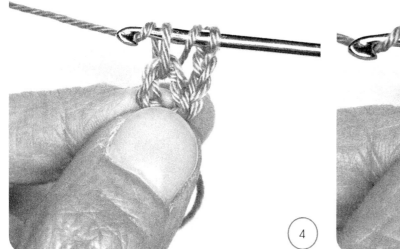

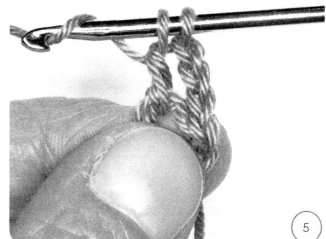

Your first double crochet is complete.

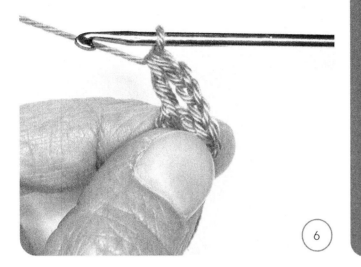

(6)

How to fasten off thread

When you reach the end of your pattern instructions cut the yarn leaving a tail about 10 inches long. Insert the tail end through the last loop left on the hook, remove the hook and pull on the tail to close the loop.
Thread the yarn tail into a yarn needle, put needle into the third chain of the first 3 chains that replace a double crochet stitch and draw yarn tail through. Fasten off by working the yarn tail into the back of your work.

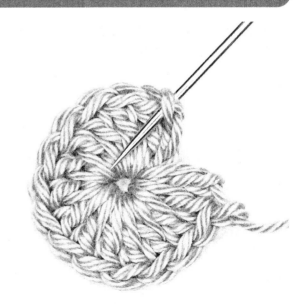

How to single crochet around rings

hold both yarn and plastic ring together properly and firmly by keeping them carefully in position as shown.

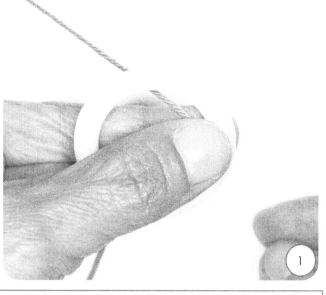

put the hook through the center of the ring.

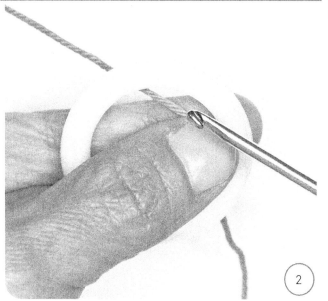

yarn over and pull up a loop (hook is now positioned above the ring).

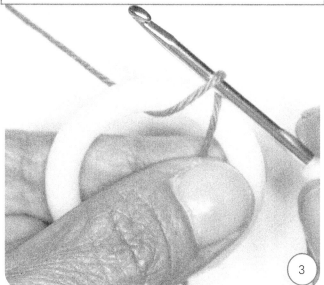

holding yarn tail firmly between yarn and forefinger, chain 1 to tighten in yarn for start off.

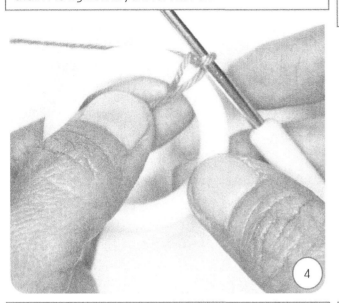

put the hook through the center of the ring and under the yarn tail, draw up a loop and make a single crochet.

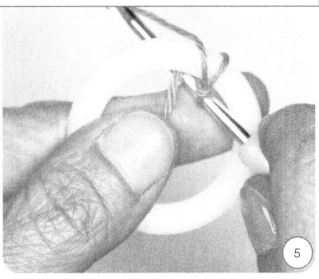

holding yarn tail firmly between yarn and forefinger continue making single crochet stitches until you have fully covered the ring, then cut the initial yarn tail.

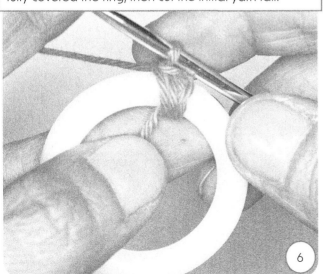

Slip stitch into the first single crochet of the round. Cut and fasten off the yarn leaving an end approx. 10 inches (25 cm) long.

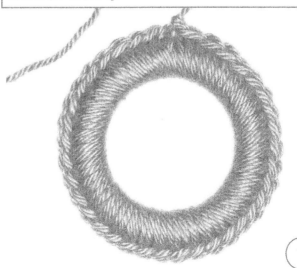

How to end each round with a slip stitch

At the end of a round, insert hook into the first stitch of that same round.

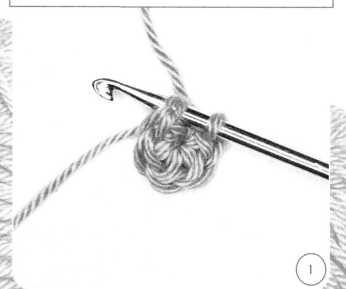

1

Make a slip stitch.

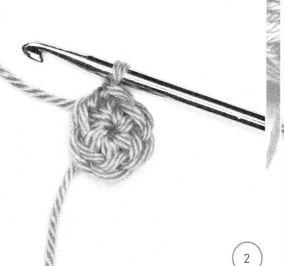

2

Chain 1, then proceed with making stitches as per pattern instructions.

3

When you reach the end of your pattern instructions, cut the yarn leaving a tail about 5 inches long.
Insert the tail end through the last loop left on the hook, remove the hook and pull on the tail to close the loop.

LET ME SHOW YOU

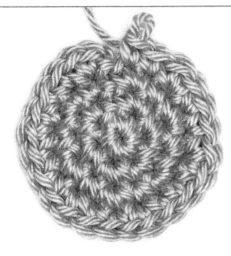

(4)

How to cut and fasten off

Thread the yarn tail into a yarn needle,

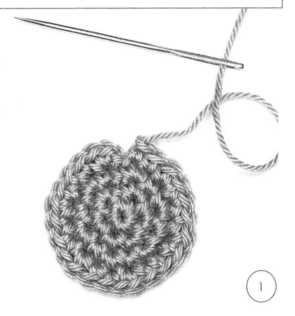

(1)

fasten off by weaving the yarn tail into the back of your work - first put needle through the 2 top loops of the 1st stitch in the round,

then weave it in and out through a couple stitches in one direction so it is invisible on the front.

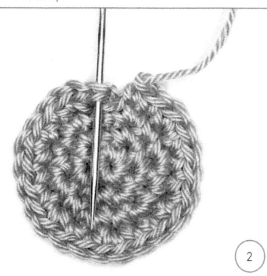

(2)

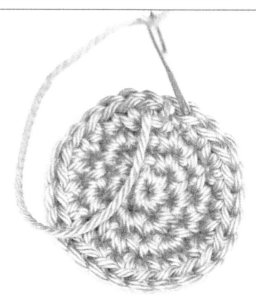

(3)

Repeat weaving in a different direction another couple of times. Cut yarn tail away flush on surface.

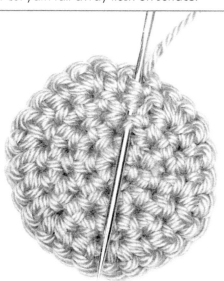

(4)

How to double crochet two together

You can double crochet 2 together into a chain ring or into the stitches of a foundation chain, a previous row or a previous round.

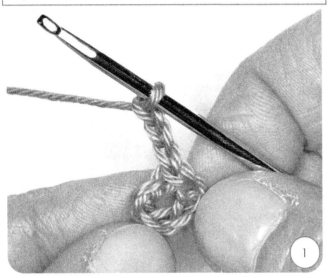

Chain 3 (this group of chains replaces your first double crochet).

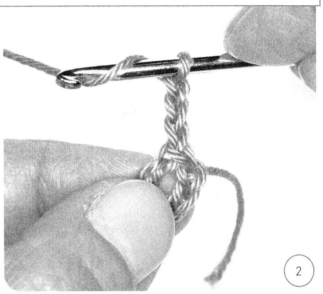

wrap yarn over hook, insert the hook into the chain ring (or into a stitch), yarn over hook again and pull up a loop back through the chain ring (or stitch).

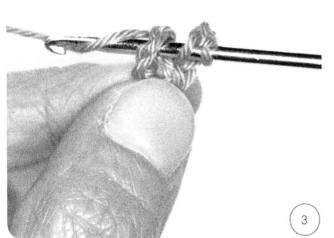

you now have 3 loops on hook. Yarn over again so you have 4 loops on hook.

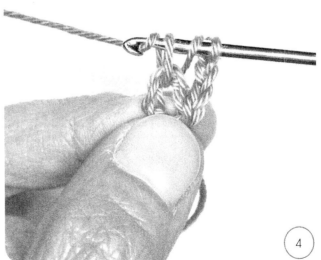

Pull through two loops, yarn over again which leaves 3 loops on hook.

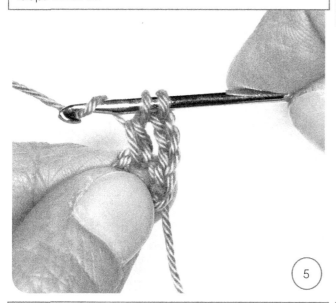

5

insert the hook into the chain ring (or into a stitch) again, yarn over hook and pull up a loop back through the chain ring (or stitch).

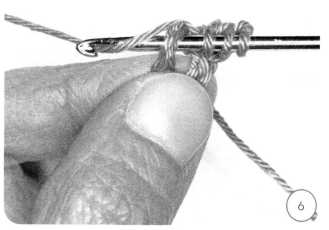

6

you now have 4 loops on hook. Yarn over again so you have 5 loops on hook.

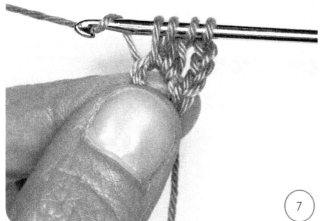

7

Pull through two loops, which leaves 3 loops on hook.

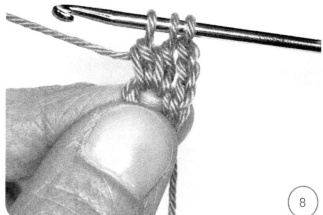

8

yarn over once more,

and pull through all 3 loops on hook, which completes the double crochet 2 together stitch.
This stitch is also known as 1 double crochet decrease.

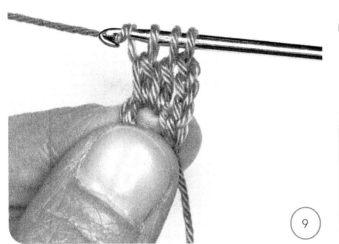

9

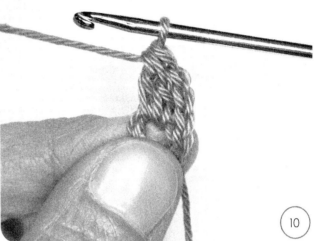

10

How to make bobble stitches

Bobble stitches are done by working a 6 double crochet cluster into the same stitch as follows:

yarn over, insert hook in stitch and pull up a loop, yarn over and pull through the first 2 loops on hook, repeat from *to* another 5 times (7 loops on hook), yarn over and pull through all loops on hook. This completes 1 bobble stitch.

Bobble stitch with a contrasting color.

With yarn color A, make a single crochet then pull up a second loop in same stitch. Holding yarn tails firmly on reverse with forefinger, wrap yarn color B around hook.

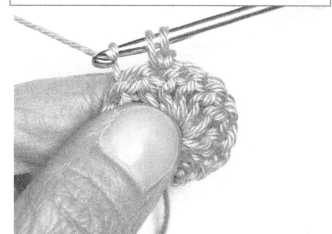

(1)

Pull color B through both loops.

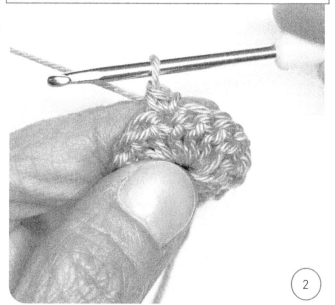

(2)

Insert hook in next stitch and make one bobble stitch with color B until you have 6 loops on hook. Holding yarn B firmly on reverse with forefinger, pull up color B from rear and wrap around hook.

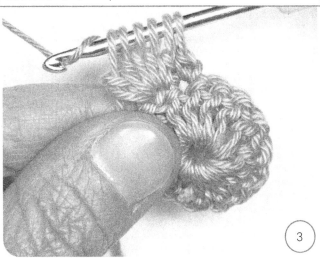

and repeat from Step 1.

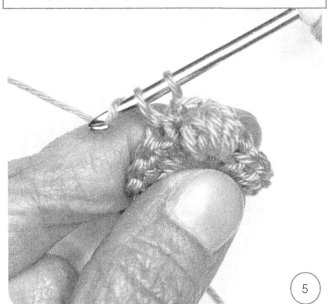

Insert hook through next stitch,

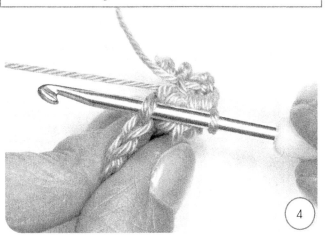

For 1 single crochet increase, work 2 sc in one stitch.
For 1 single crochet decrease, close
2 single crochet stitches together as follows: insert hook and draw up a loop in each of the next two stitches so that there are 3 loops on hook, yarn over and draw through all 3 loops together. This is also known as a "single crochet 2 together" stitch.

NOTE: When instructed to begin each round or each row with ch 1, this ch simply serves to start off a single crochet round or row and will not substitute a stitch. Unless you are given other instructions, simply ignore and skip it, both when ending the round (or row) and when starting off the next round (or row).
When instructed to begin each round or each row with ch 3, these ch simply serve to start off a double crochet round or row and will not substitute a stitch. Unless you are given other instructions, simply ignore and skip them, both when ending the round (or row) and when starting off the next round (or row).

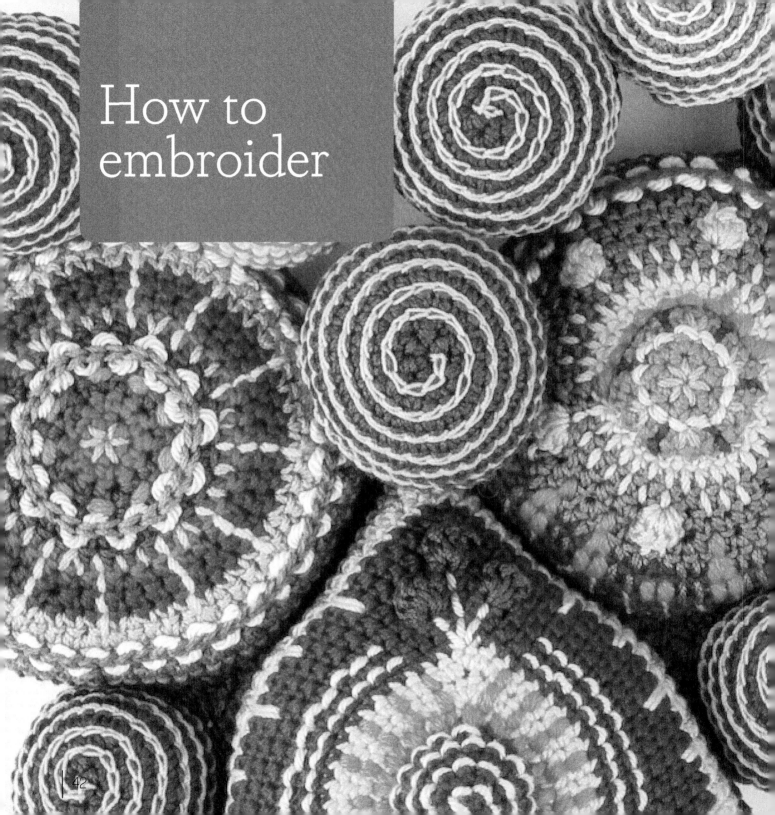

How to embroider

Embroidery can unexpectedly and radically change the appearance of your crochet fabric.

You have two ways of making embroidered embellishments:

you can either embroider in a circle, working around the spaces between rounds, e.g. in the gaps between rounds 1 and 2;

or you can embroider in straight lines, working from the center or from the base of your piece and then up through the stitch-gaps of each stitch built above the last.

The pictures below and on the previous page show some crochet balls embroidered with rounds of chain stitches.

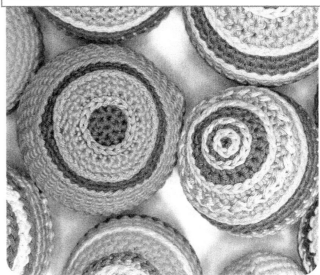

You can use any type and weight of yarn, although it is best to select a yarn that is heavier than the yarn used for your crochet piece, especially when embroidering basic stitches. My advice to you is: use your leftover yarn scraps!

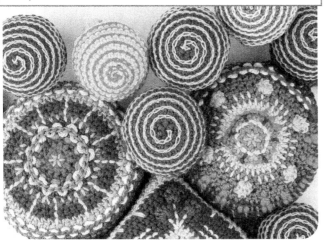

SUPER TIP: I generally embroider on the back surface of my crochet work because I think it's easier to identify the stitches, the stitch-gaps and the gaps between the rounds. I suggest you try the same!

Thread your yarn needle with a length of yarn, leave the shorter end open and make an overhand knot on the longer end. Always start by bringing your needle out of your work at the starting point from behind and pulling on your yarn gently until the knot is blocked up against the rear and stops the yarn pulling right through. If the yarn does pull through, make a double overhand knot.

Straight stitch embroidery in a circle
Bring your needle out at the starting point, then *put your yarn needle into the first stitch-gap located backwards right, then bring it out of the stitch-gap located one gap away to the left*; repeat from *to*.

Chain stitch embroidery in a circle
This is done with the front surface of your work (right side) facing you:
bring your needle out at the starting point from behind, then *holding the yarn to the left of your needle, put the needle back into the starting point and bring it out through the next stitch-gap without pulling it out completely, loop the yarn around under the needle from left to right then pull the needle out completely to tighten the loop that has formed. Put your needle back into the same stitch-gap but from inside the loop*; repeat from * to *.

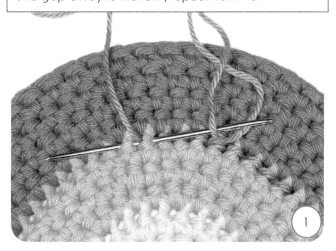

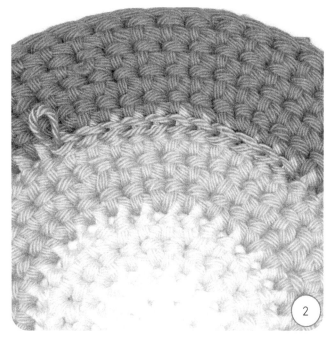

Straight stitch embroidery in a straight line
Bring your needle out at the starting point, then *put your yarn needle into the gap between rounds upwards from the starting point, then bring it out of the gap located in the next round upwards*; repeat from *to*.

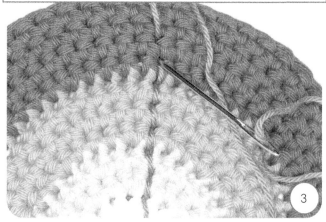

Chain stitch embroidery in a straight line
This is done with the front surface of your work (right side) facing you:

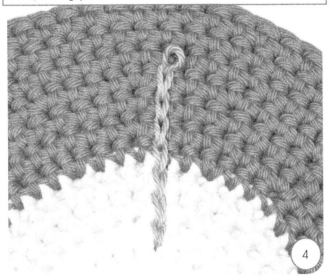

bring your needle out at the starting point from behind, then *holding the yarn to the left of your needle,

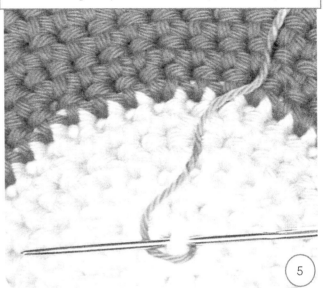

put the needle back into the starting point and bring it out of the gap located in the next round upwards without pulling it out completely, loop the yarn around under the needle from left to right then pull the needle out completely to tighten the loop that has formed. Put your needle back into the same gap but from inside the loop*; repeat from * to *.

You can work chain stitches on the front surface of your work either using a yarn needle as instructed, or you can also do so using a crochet hook.
In this case the stitch is called "surface crochet slip stitch".
To make surface crochet slip stitches, the yarn is held against the back surface of the fabric by the non-working hand while the hook is held along the front surface by the working hand.

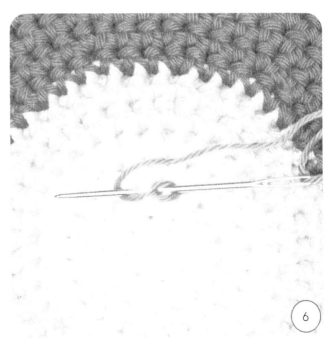

Make a slip knot and hold it in place against the back surface of the crochet fabric directly under the starting point,
*insert hook into crocheted fabric from front to back, pick up slip knot with hook and pull slip knot loop through to the front.

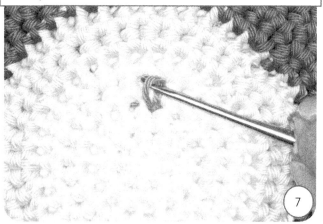

Insert hook again from front to back (either through the next stitch-gap or through the gap located in the next round upwards),

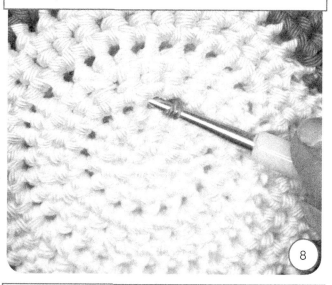

pull up a second loop to the front side (picture here shows back of work),

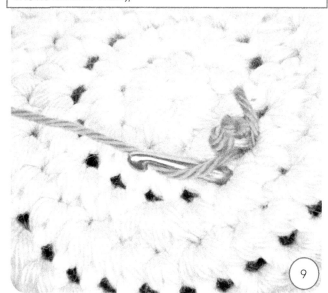

and pull this second loop through the first loop in one motion*.
Repeat from * to *.

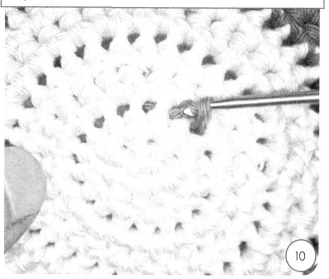

How to close an embroidery stitch round

Thread yarn tail in through first stich from top to bottom.

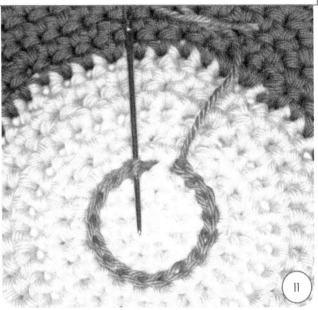

Put needle in through middle of first stitch, from front to back, then fasten off yarn tail on reverse.

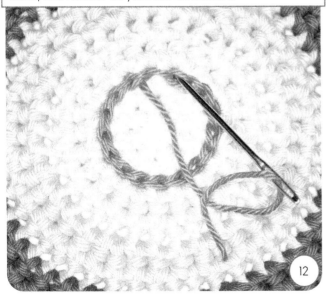

How to embroider woven stitches

Woven embroidery stitches are used to embellish basic embroidery stitches and are usually done in a contrasting color.

Step 13

To embroider woven straight stitches (or woven chain stitches), *bring your needle out at the starting point from the beginning of a straight stitch (or of a chain stitch), then weave your needle in through the next stitch from right to left,

gently pulling on the yarn until you have a small loop to the side.

Step 14

Next, weave your needle in through the following stitch from left to right leaving a small loop on the opposite side*.

While weaving in and out, your needle must not touch the fabric - make sure you only pass through the yarn.

Step 15

Repeat from * - * for all the woven stitches you want to make.

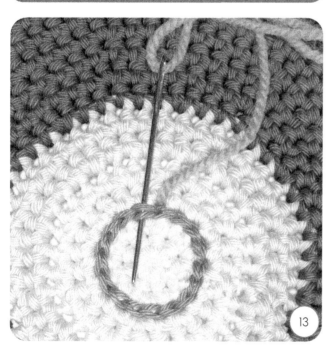

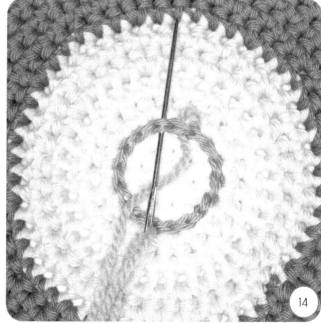

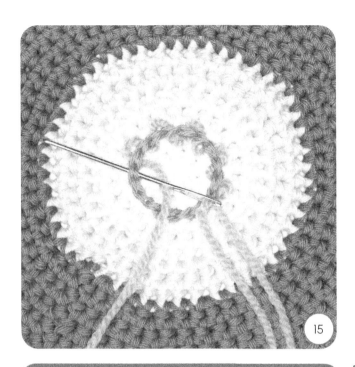

Bullion knot stitch

Bring your needle out at the starting point without pulling it out completely, wind the thread around the needle about 5 times and holding the thread coils in place with your thumb, finish pulling the needle through and put it back in about 1 mm away from the starting point. Pull needle and thread completely out from the back of your work very gently for a good, even formation of the bullion knot on the surface.

LET ME SHOW YOU

How to make round 3d crochet elements

Each round 3D crochet element is made up of 2 sections crocheted separately
(front and rear or top and bottom) that are then joined together in the course of the project.

When sewing or crocheting the two sections of the round 3D elements together, remember to leave a large enough opening for filling. To do so, roll a sufficient amount of fiber fill or toy stuffing into a small, tight ball and place it inside the 2 sections through the opening. Cut and fasten off yarn.

#1 How to crochet two round element sections together

Step 1
Make 2 identical polka dots (section 1 and section 2). When section 1 is complete, cut and fasten off yarn.

Step 2
At the end of the last round of section 2 do not cut yarn but end with a sl st . Place back of section 2 against back of section 1 with stitches of last rounds matching up together, *insert hook into both the next stitch of section 2 and directly into the corresponding stitch of section 1, pull up a loop through both sections, yarn over and pull through both loops to sc 1*. Repeat to join all stitches round.

Step 3
Remember to leave a large enough opening for filling with either fiber-fill or toy stuffing.

Step 4
Cut and fasten off yarn.

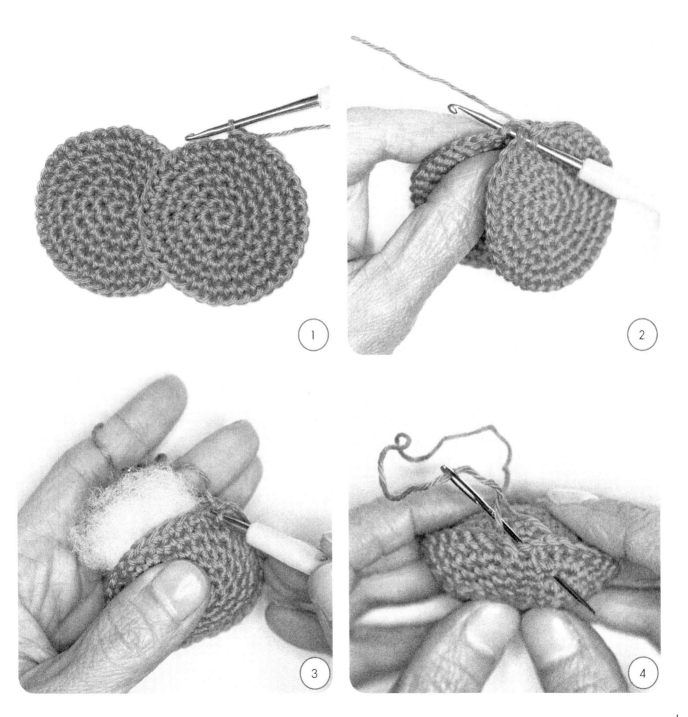

#2 How to sew two round element sections together with a decorative embroidery stitch: the scroll stitch.

Step 5

Make 2 identical polka dots (section 1 and section 2), cut and fasten off yarn on both sections. Hold back surfaces of both sections against one another with stitches of last rounds matching up together.

With a yarn needle and a length of yarn that is heavier than the yarn used for your polka dots, bring needle out at starting point then put needle in from front to back through both the stitch of the section facing you and the corresponding stitch in the section behind it, without pulling it out completely.

Step 6

Pull the working yarn frontwards and then completely around the needle in a circular motion from front to back.

Step 7

Gently pull the needle out completely so that the yarn tightens into a circular knot.

Step 8

Put needle in from front to back through the next stitch along in the section facing you and the corresponding stitch in the section behind it, without pulling it out completely, repeat Steps 6 and 7.

Repeat * to * to join all stitches round, minding that you leave a large enough opening for filling.

Cut and fasten off yarn.

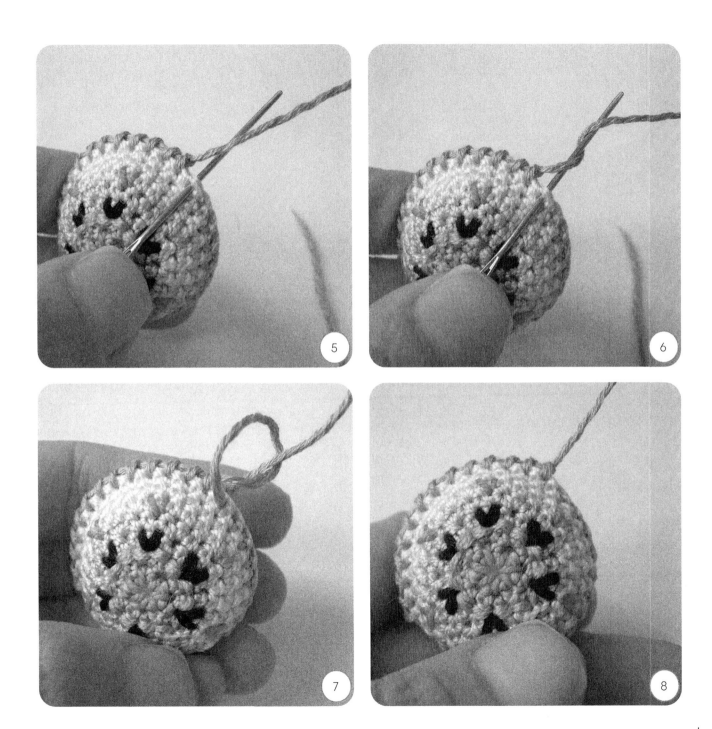

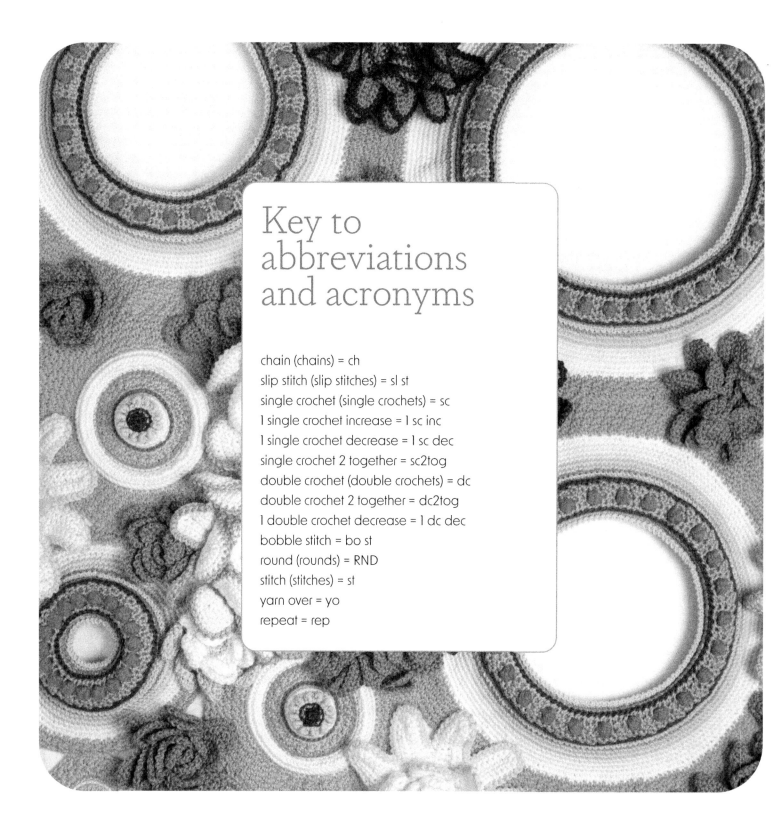

Key to abbreviations and acronyms

chain (chains) = ch
slip stitch (slip stitches) = sl st
single crochet (single crochets) = sc
1 single crochet increase = 1 sc inc
1 single crochet decrease = 1 sc dec
single crochet 2 together = sc2tog
double crochet (double crochets) = dc
double crochet 2 together = dc2tog
1 double crochet decrease = 1 dc dec
bobble stitch = bo st
round (rounds) = RND
stitch (stitches) = st
yarn over = yo
repeat = rep

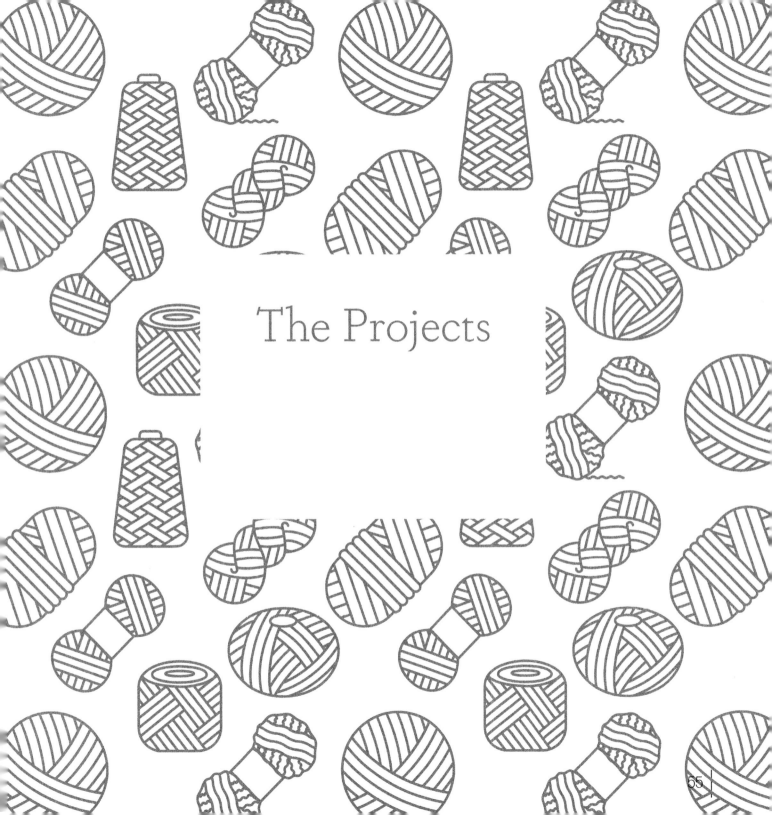

The Projects

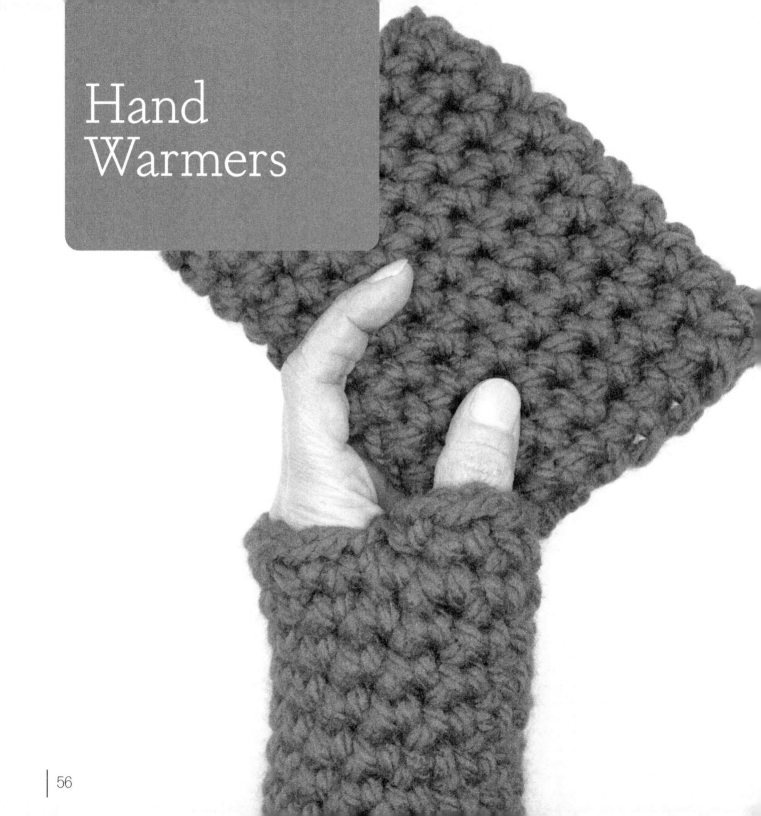

Hand
Warmers

Hand Warmers

MATERIALS

100% acrylic | super bulky (6) weight yarn (3.5oz = 65.5yds / 100g = 60m) | color: indigo
crochet hook size N/P-15 (10 mm)
yarn needle

PATTERN STITCHES

ch, sl st, sc

INSTRUCTIONS

Make a foundation chain as long as needed to fit the circumference of your hand at its widest point.
Insert hook into the first foundation ch, sc 1 into each of the following chains then continue working in a continuous spiral (never joining rounds). When your work reaches your required hand size, end with a sl st. Cut and fasten off yarn.
Slip the warmer onto your hand, mark the thumb hole size along the top edge and sew as illustrated.
Make 2!

SUPER TIP

For smoother insertion of hook in round 1, make the foundation chain using a size P-16 hook, then proceed working the sc stitches with the N/P-15 hook. While crocheting, don't pull on your yarn too tightly – this will help to give your fabric a nice, soft drape.

LET ME SHOW YOU

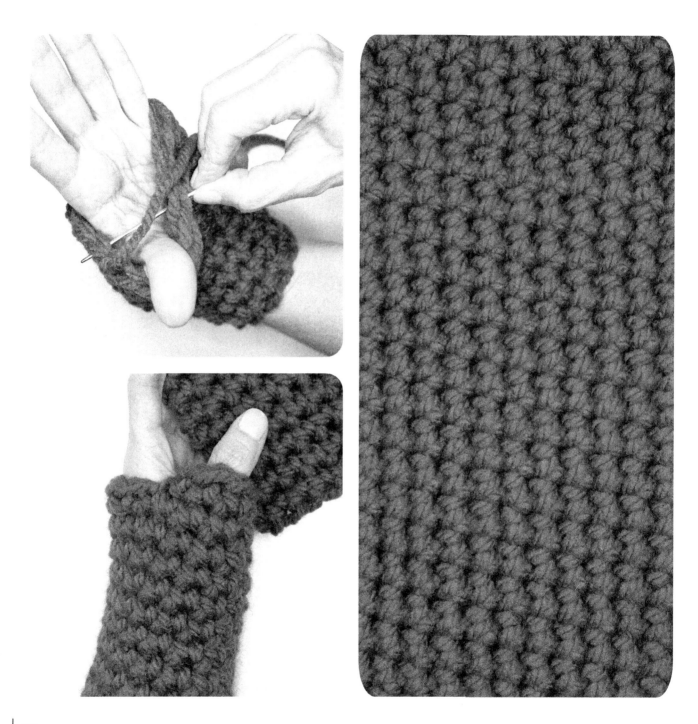

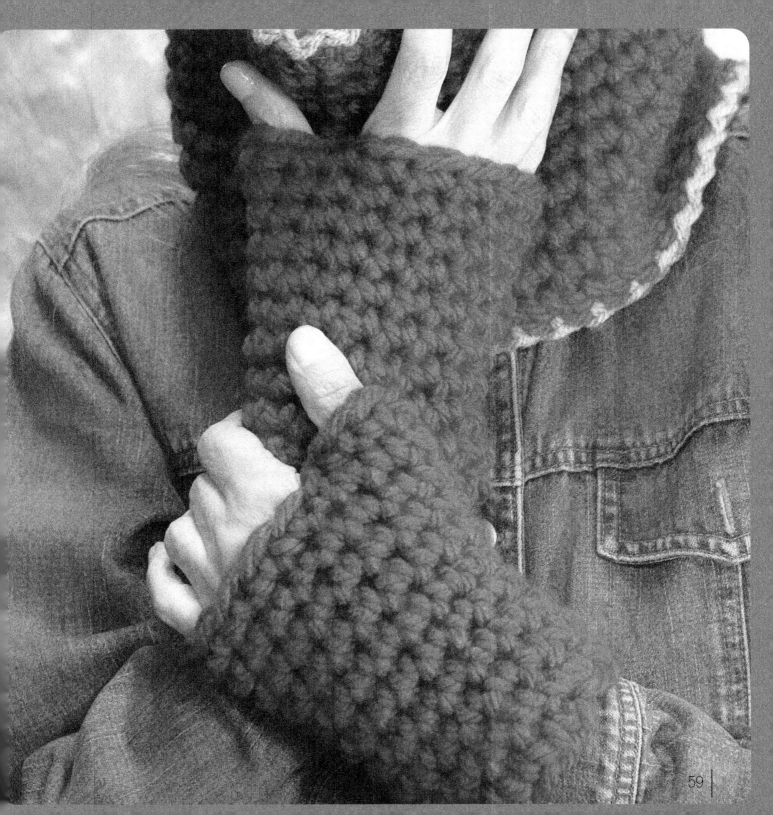

Fitted Neck Warmer

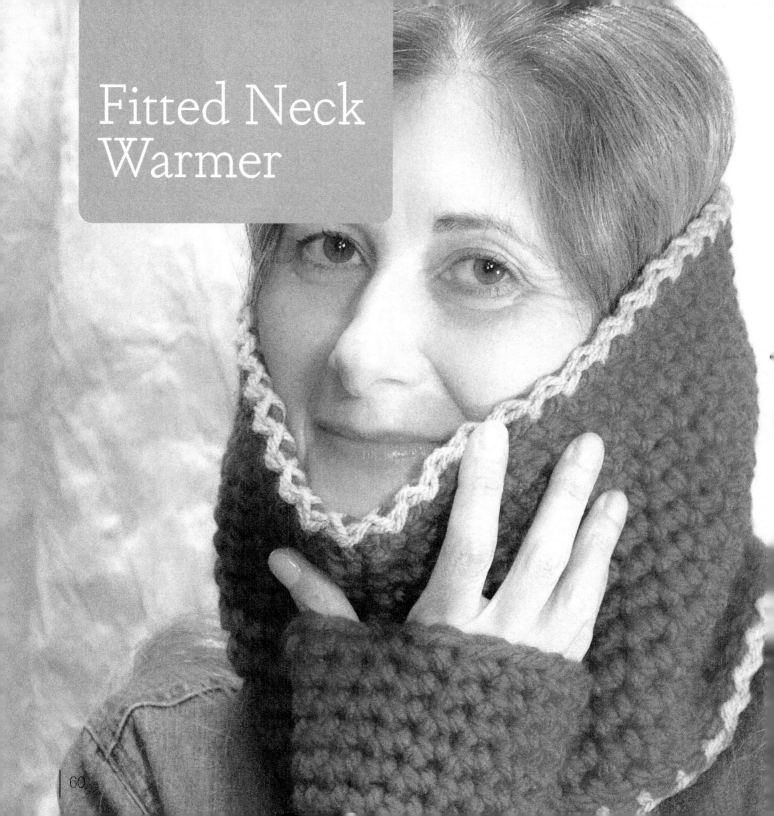

Fitted Neck Warmer

MATERIALS

100% acrylic | super bulky (6) weight yarn (3.5oz = 65.5yds / 100g = 60m) | color: burgundy
crochet hook size N/P-15 (10 mm)
100% acrylic | bulky (5) weight yarn (3.5oz = 180yds / 100g = 165m) | color: light pink
crochet hook size I-9 (5.50 mm)
yarn needle

PATTERN STITCHES

ch, sl st, sc

INSTRUCTIONS

With the burgundy yarn and your size N/P-15 hook, ch 40. Now follow the same instructions given for the hand warmers until you count about 14 rounds. End with a sl st, cut and fasten off yarn.

With the light pink yarn and your size I-9 hook, insert hook into any one of the stitches along the top row, ch 1 to fasten on yarn. Then *sl st 1 and ch1 in next stitch*; rep from *to* to the end of the round, ss 1 to close round. Cut and fasten off yarn. Next, ch 1 to fasten the light pink yarn into any one of the foundation chains, rep from *to* to the end of the round, ss 1 to close round then cut and fasten off yarn.

LET ME SHOW YOU

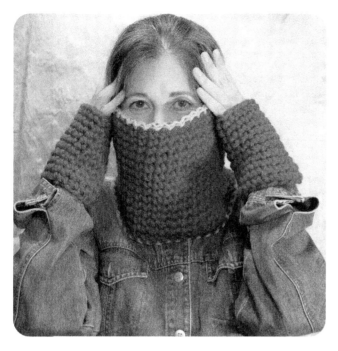

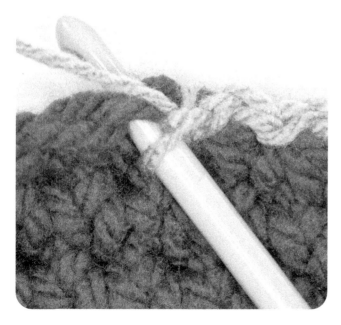

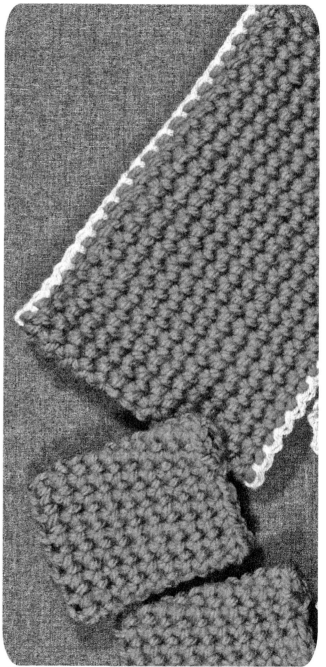

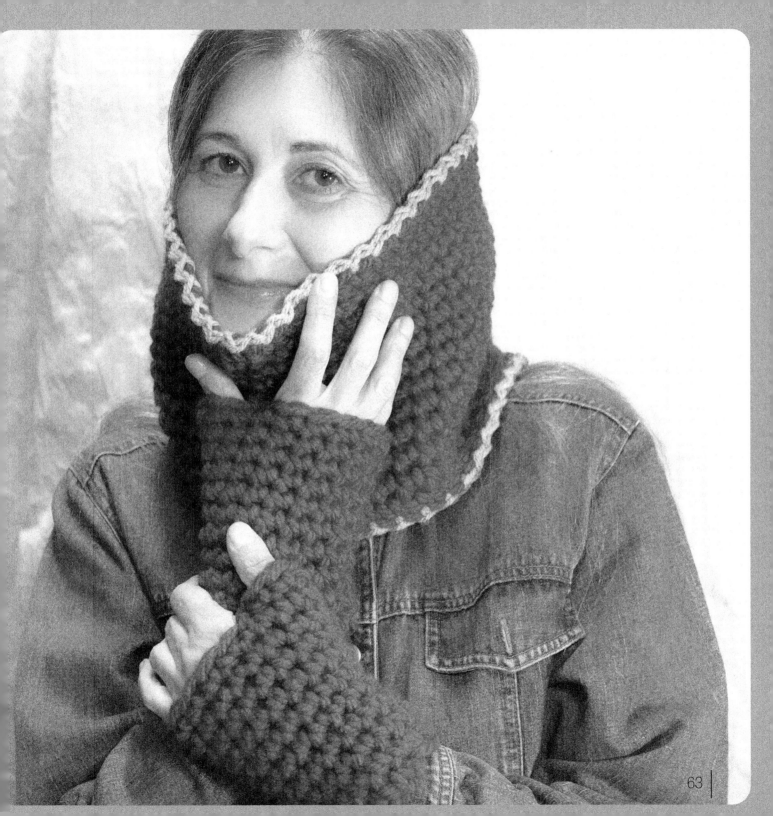

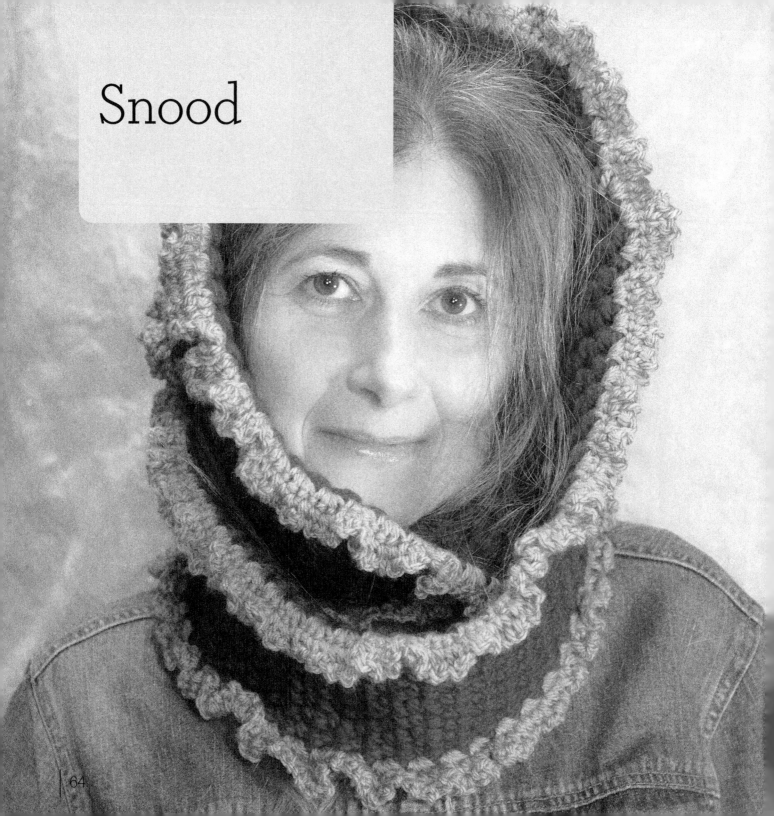

Snood

Snood

MATERIALS

100% acrylic | super bulky (6) weight yarn (7oz = 131yds /
200g = 120m) | color: royal blue
crochet hook size N/P-15 (10 mm)
100% acrylic | bulky (5) weight yarn (3.5oz = 180yds /
100g = 165m) | color: celadon green
crochet hook size I-9 (5.50 mm)
yarn needle

PATTERN STITCHES

ch, sl st, sc

INSTRUCTIONS

With the royal blue yarn and your size N/P-15 hook, ch
80.
Check to ensure that the chain does not twist on itself and,
holding it straight, insert hook into the first foundation ch,
sc 1, then sc 1 into each of the following foundation chains.
Continue working in a continuous spiral (never joining
rounds) till you reach the end of the skein. End with a sl st,
cut and work in yarn end.

With the celadon green yarn and your size I-9 hook,
work as follows
RND 1: insert hook into any one of the stitches along
the top row, ch 1 to fasten in yarn then sc 3 in each stitch
around.
RND 2: *sc 1, ch 2* in first st of new round, rep from *to* to
the end of the round, cut and fasten off yarn.
Next, ch 1 to fasten the celadon green yarn into any one
of the foundation chains, rep as done for RND 1 and RND
2 above on this side too. Cut and fasten off thread.

LET ME SHOW YOU

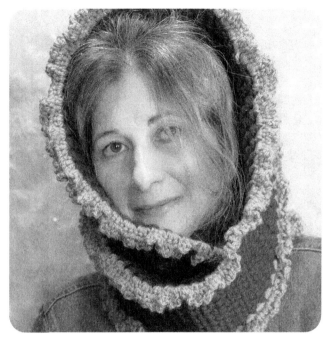

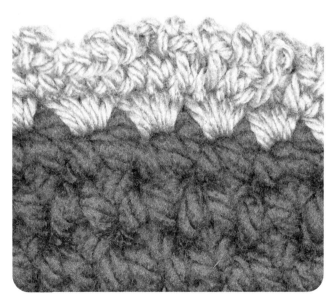

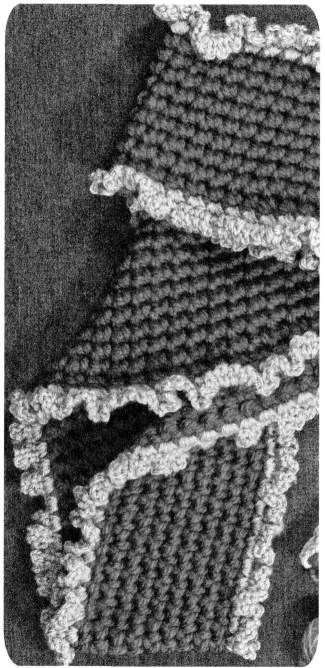

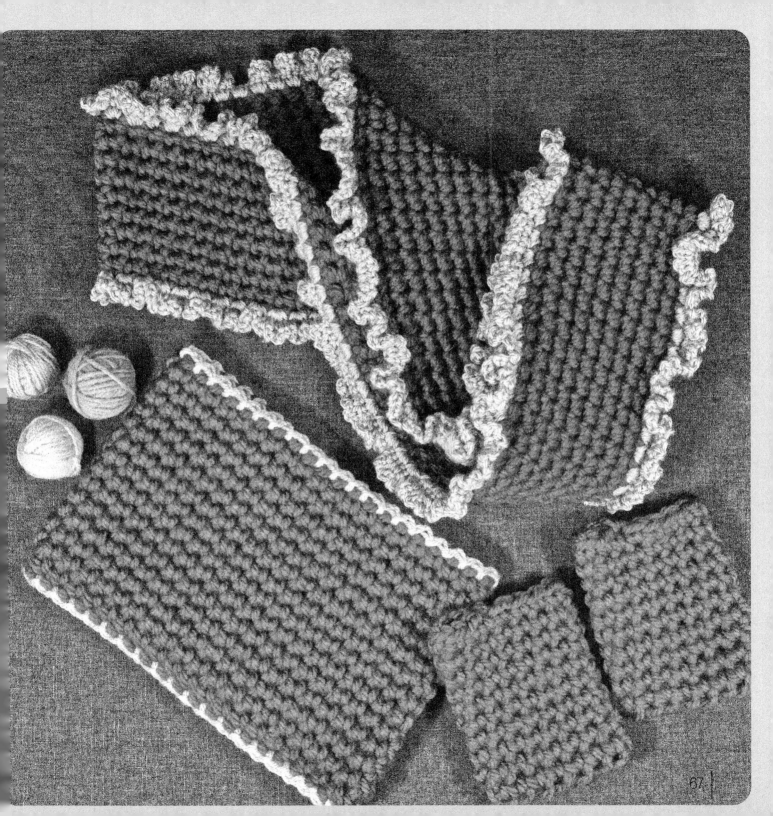

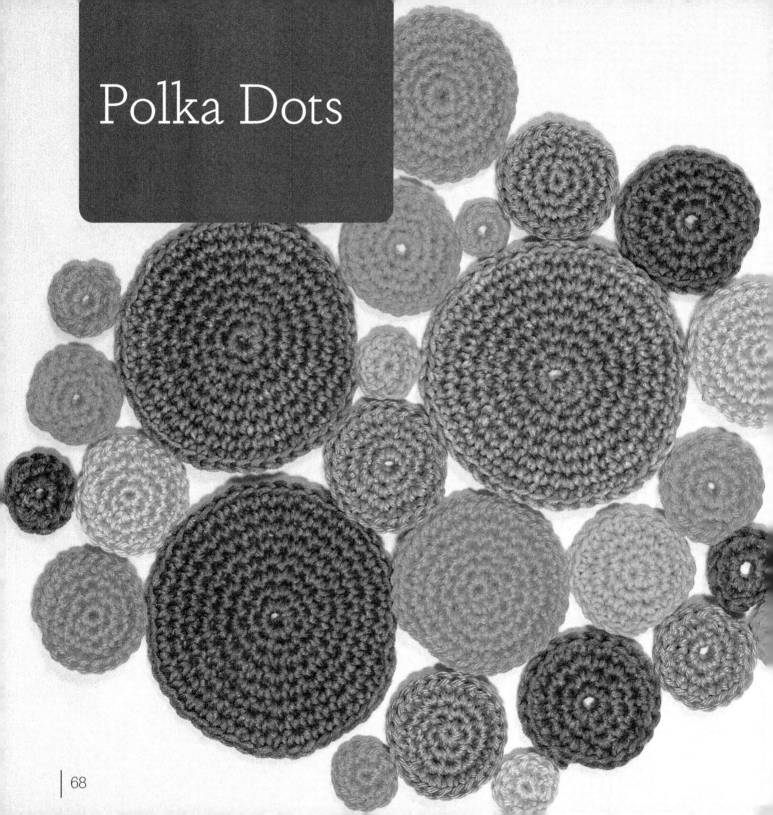

Polka Dots

Polka Dots

EXTRA SMALL, SMALL, MEDIUM AND LARGE POLKA DOTS

With these flat, circular, disk-like crochet elements we will practice doing increases using stitch markers to keep track of your rounds.

You'll learn to make circular elements in a range of different sizes and to mix them together for multiple uses, such as the creation of original fashion and home-decor accessories.

Try to follow the step by step instructions as accurately as possible, remembering to count the number of stitches done in each round and then to compare it with the number of stitches stated in brackets on the pattern to check whether you have the right number of stitches or not.

Insert a stitch marker into the first stitch of each round and remember to move it up when starting the next round.

Stay relaxed while crocheting: these projects are designed so that they don't necessarily have to be one hundred percent perfect. If you find that at the end of a round you haven't worked in the right number of increases and you end up with a few stitches more or a few less, don't worry! Keep going and do your best to keep your fabric flat by crocheting in a continuous spiral and by working in a regular number of increases. Start practicing by making at least 5 extra small, 5 small and 5 medium polka dots and, when you feel confident, move on to larger circles.

SUPER TIP: once you have the size you require, sl st 1 in next stitch to end round, cut yarn and fasten off. If you plan instead to attach or sew the circle into a project, before cutting your yarn leave a long enough tail which should go from a minimum of about 12" to a maximum of about 18" long.

LET ME SHOW YOU

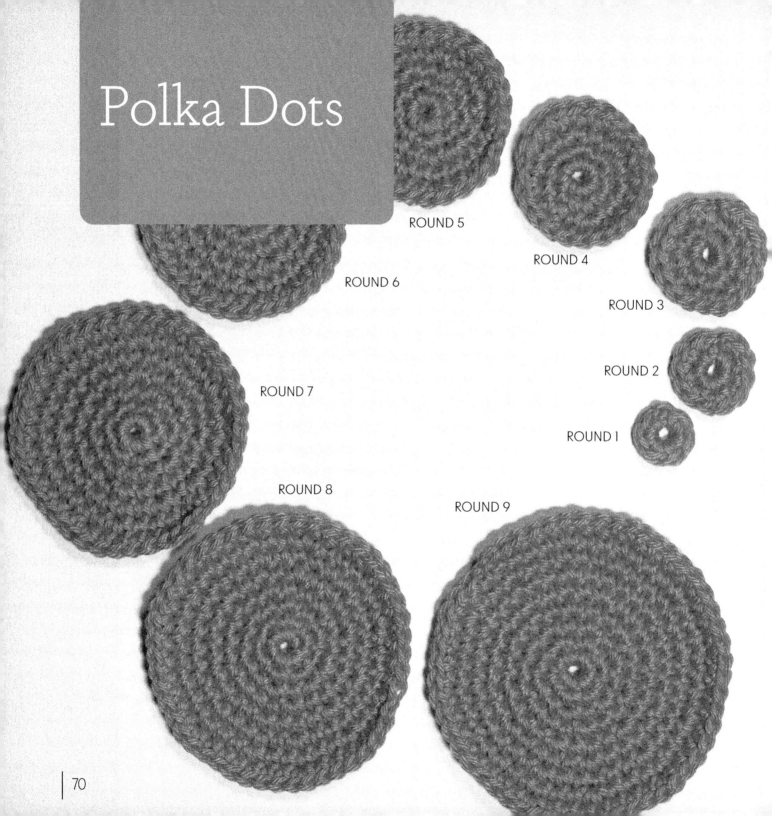

Polka Dots

ROUND 5

ROUND 6

ROUND 4

ROUND 3

ROUND 7

ROUND 2

ROUND 1

ROUND 8

ROUND 9

Polka Dots

MATERIALS

Choose solid color yarns (and/or gradient colors and/or radial-gradient colored yarns) to your own personal liking, suitable for the crochet hook size you intend using
yarn needle
1 stitch marker

PATTERN STITCHES

ch, sl st, sc

STEP BY STEP INSTRUCTIONS

STEP 1

Ch 4, sl st 1 into the first ch to form a loop.
RND 1: ch 1, sc 6.

STEP 2

RND 2: *sc 2 in each stitch*, rep from *to* another 5 times (12 stitches).

STEP 3

RND 3: *sc 1, sc 2 in the following stitch (1 increase)*; rep from *to* another 5 times (18 stitches).

STEP 4

RND 4: *sc 2 in next stitch (1 increase), sc 1 in following 2 stitches*; rep from *to* another 5 times (24 stitches).

STEP 5

RND 5: *sc 1 into each of the following 3 stitches, sc 2 into the next stitch (1 increase)* rep from *to* another 5 times (30 stitches).

STEP 6

RND 6: sc 1, *sc 2 into the next stitch (1 increase), sc 1 into

each of the following 4 stitches*, rep from *to* another 5 times (36 stitches).

STEP 7

RND 7 : *sc 1 into each of the following 5 stitches, sc 2 into the next stitch (1 increase)* rep from *to* another 5 times (42 stitches).

STEP 8

RND 8: sc 1 into each of the following 2 stitches, *sc 2 into the next stitch (1 increase), sc 1 into each of the following 4 stitches*, rep from *to* another 5 times (48 stitches).

STEP 9

RND 9: *sc 1 into each of the following 7 stitches, sc 2 into the next stitch (1 increase)* rep *to* for another 5 times (54 stitches).

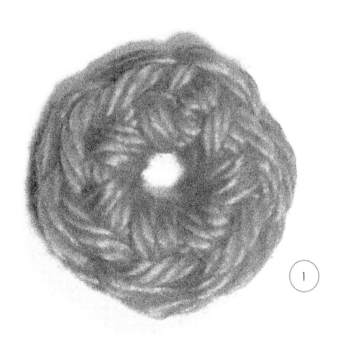

(1)

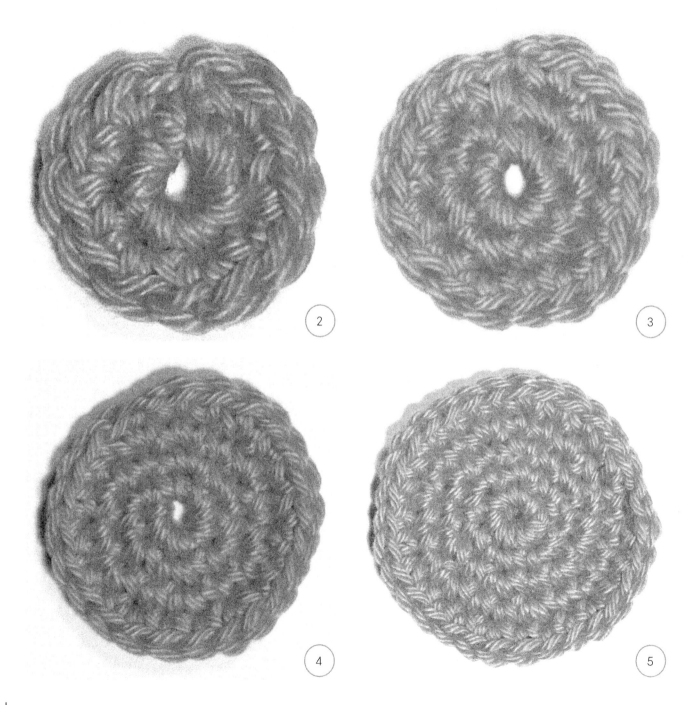

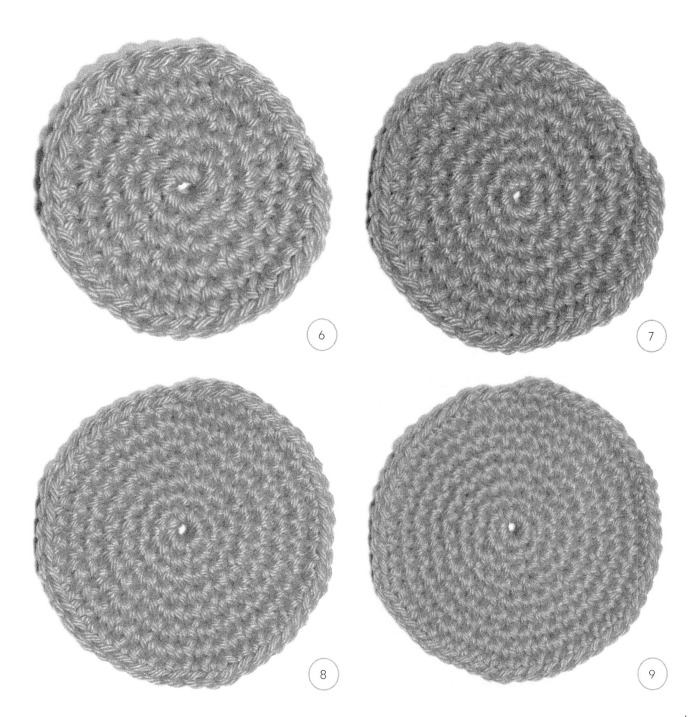

Extra Large Crochet Circle

Extra Large Crochet Circle

MATERIALS

3.5 oz (100 g) of gradient colored and/or radial-gradient colored light (3) weight yarn
crochet hook size E-4 (3.50 mm)
yarn needle
1 stitch marker

PATTERN STITCHES

ch, sl st, sc

INSTRUCTIONS

For an extra large crochet circle (having a diameter of approx. 9"), follow the instructions given for the largest polka dot, but do not cut yarn and fasten off after round 9. Continue building on more rounds as follows:

RND 10: sc 1 into each of the following 3 stitches, *sc 2 into the next stitch (1 increase), sc 1 into each of the following 5 stitches*, rep from *to* another 5 times (60 stitches).

RND 11: sc 1 into each stitch around (60 stitches).

RND 12: *sc 2 in next stitch (1 increase), sc 1 in following 2 stitches*; rep from *to* another 19 times (80 stitches).

RND 13 and 14: sc 1 into each stitch around (80 stitches).

RND 15: *sc 1 into each of the following 3 stitches, sc 2 into the next stitch (1 increase)* rep from *to* another 19 times (100 stitches).

RND 16, 17 and 18: sc 1 into each stitch around (100 stitches).

RND 19: sc 1, *sc 2 into the next stitch (1 increase), sc 1 into each of the following 4 stitches*, rep from *to* another 19 times (120 stitches).

RND 20, 21, 22 and 23: sc 1 into each stitch around (120 stitches), sl st 1 to close round.

Cut yarn and fasten off.

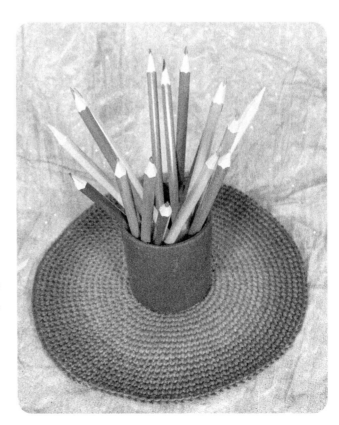

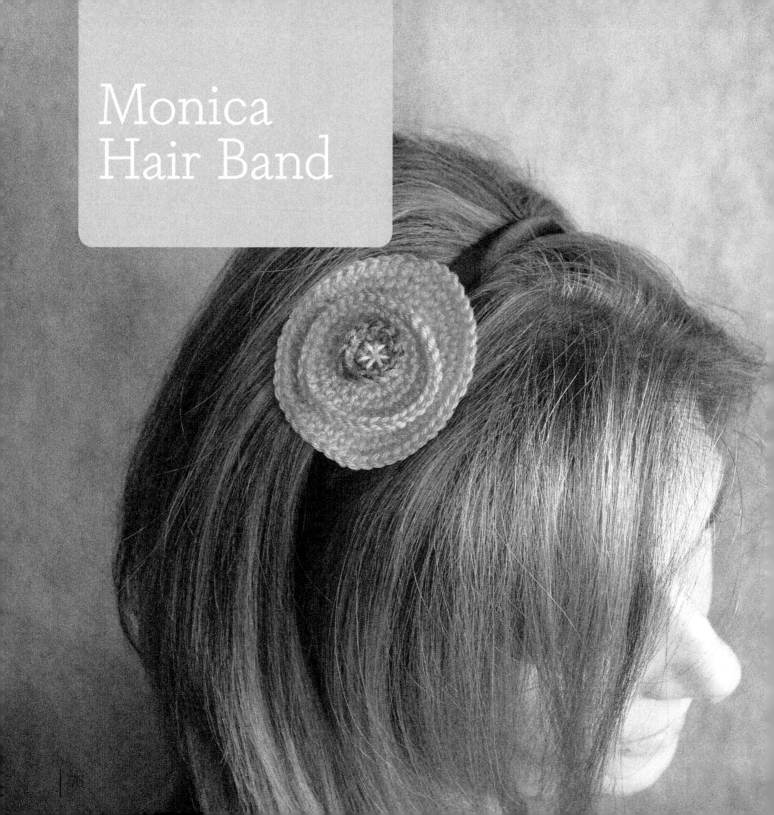

Monica Hair Band

Monica Hair Band

This hair band decoration is formed by 3 round disk elements crocheted separately and then sewn together.

MATERIALS

100% cotton | fine (2) weight yarn (1.75oz = 137yds / 50g = 125m)

about half an oz (about 15 g) in each of the following colors: fuchsia, lobster red, light blue;

about 8" (20 cm) are additionally required in bright yellow

crochet hook C-2 or D-3 (3.25 – 3.75 mm)

yarn needle

1 hairband

PATTERN STITCHES

ch, sl st, sc

LET ME SHOW YOU

INSTRUCTIONS

Small element a

With the light blue form a double loop and insert hook,

RND 1: ch 1, sc 6.

RND 2: *sc 2 in each stitch*, rep from *to* another 5 times (12 stitches).

Sl st 1 to close round, cut yarn and fasten off.

Medium element a

With the fuchsia follow the instructions given for the small element a, at the end of round 2 do not cut yarn but proceed as follows:

RND 3: *sc 1, sc 2 in the following stitch (1 increase)*; rep from *to* another 5 times (18 stitches).

RND 4: *sc 2 in first stitch (1 increase), sc 1 in following 2 stitches*; rep from *to* another 5 times (24 stitches).

RND 5: *sc 1 into each of the following 3 stitches, sc 2 into the next stitch (1 increase)* rep from *to* another 5 times (30 stitches).

Sl st 1 to close round, cut yarn and fasten off.

Large element a

With the lobster red follow the instructions given for the medium element a, at the end of round 5 do not cut yarn but proceed as follows:

RND 6: sc 1, *sc 2 into the next stitch (1 increase), sc 1 into each of the following 4 stitches*, rep from *to* another 5 times (36 stitches).

RND 7: *sc 1 into each of the following 5 stitches, sc 2 into the next stitch (1 increase)* rep from *to* another 5 times (42 stitches).

Sl st 1 to close round, cut yarn and fasten off.

Overlap the three round elements as illustrated and sew them so that they are held together with straight stitches going from the center of the small round element into the spaces between the top of each sc in the first round, to form a star.

Sew the decoration into position onto the hair band

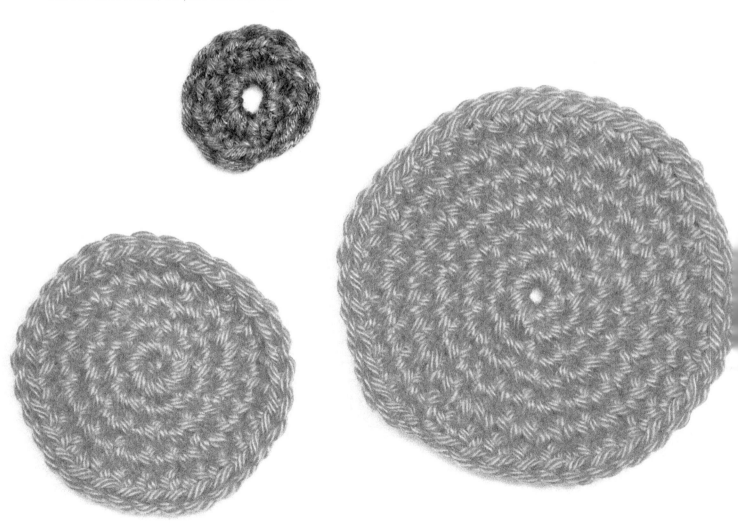

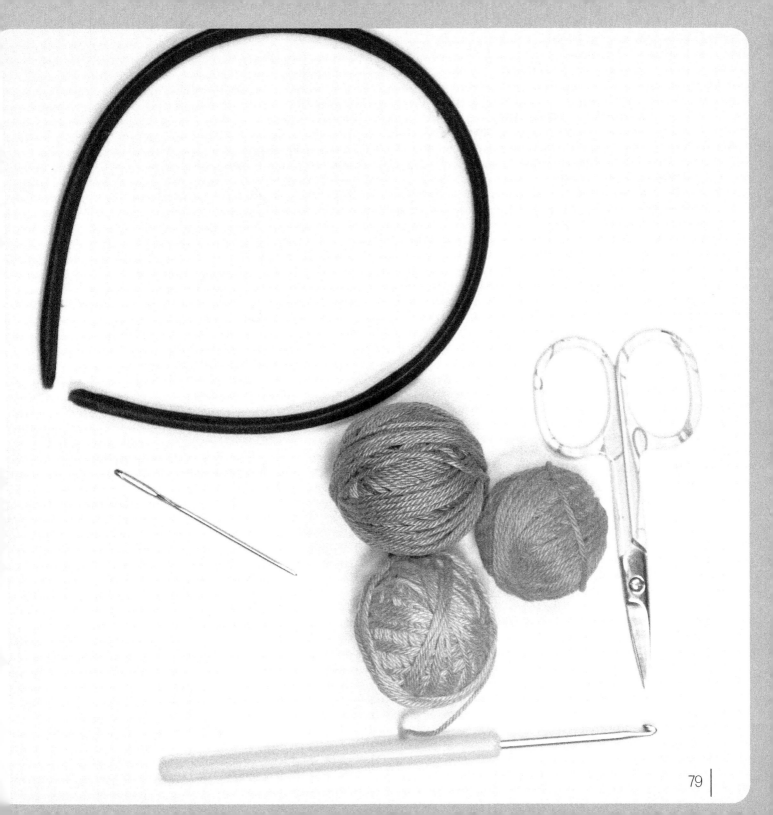

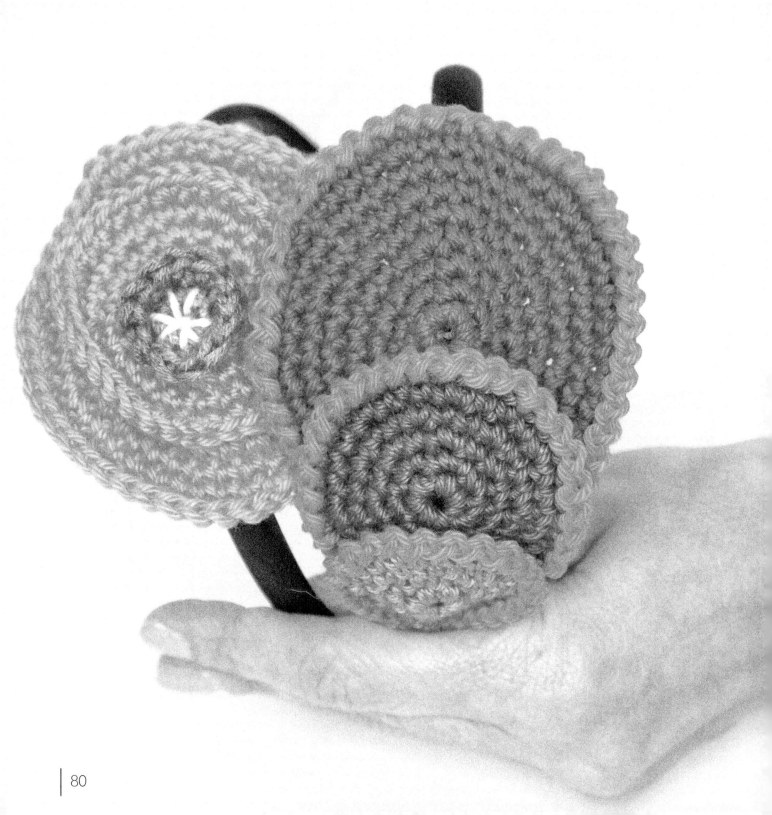

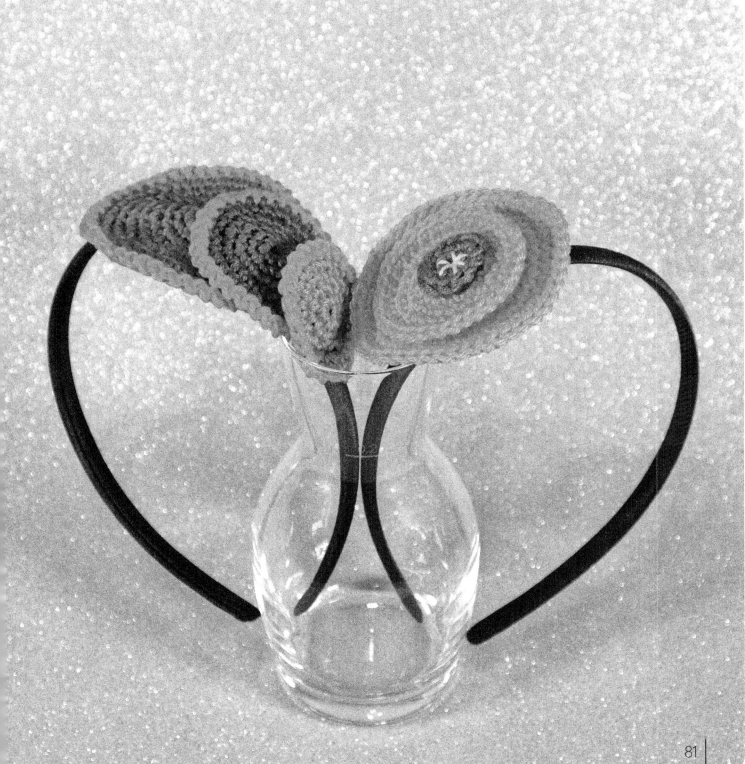

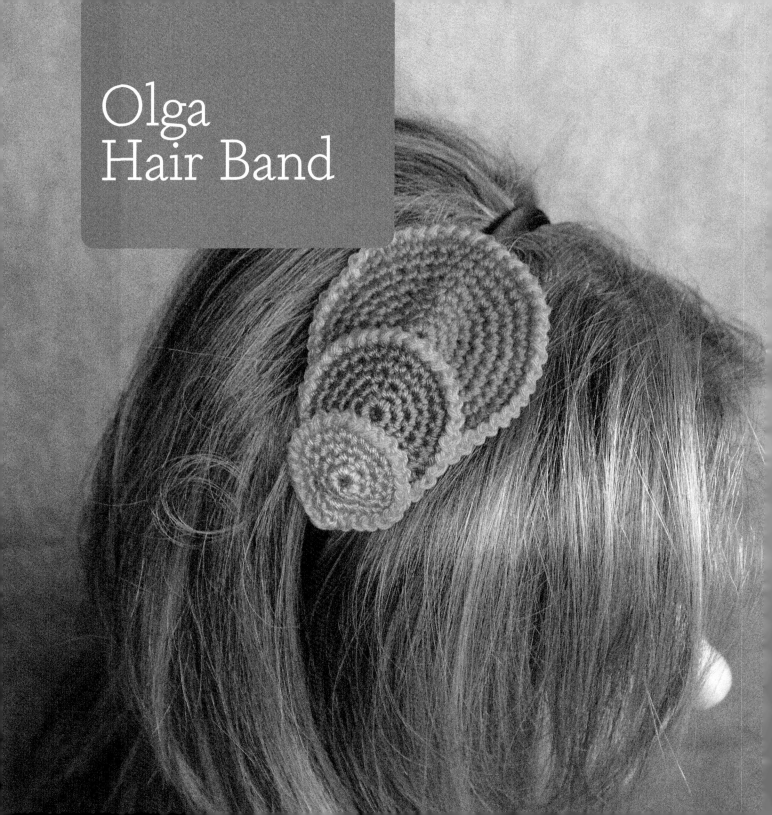

Olga
Hair Band

Olga Hair Band

This hair band decoration is formed by 3 round disk elements crocheted separately and then sewn together.

MATERIALS

100% cotton | fine (2) weight yarn (1.75oz = 137yds / 50g = 125m)
about half an oz (about 15 g) in each of the following colors: burgundy, purple, cyclamen purple and orange
crochet hook C-2 or D-3 (3.25 – 3.75 mm)
yarn needle
1 hairband

PATTERN STITCHES

ch, sl st, sc

INSTRUCTIONS

Small element b

With the cyclamen purple form a double loop and insert hook
RND 1: ch 1, sc 6.

LET ME SHOW YOU

RND 2: *sc 2 in each stitch*, rep from *to* another 5 times (12 stitches).
RND 3: *sc 1, sc 2 in the following stitch (1 increase)*; rep from *to* another 5 times (18 stitches).
RND 4: *sc 2 in next stitch (1 increase), sc 1 in following 2 stitches*; rep from *to* another 5 times (24 stitches).
Sl st 1 to close round, cut yarn and fasten off.

Medium element b

With the purple follow the instructions given for the small round element at the end of round 4 do not cut yarn but proceed as follows:
RND 5: *sc 1 into each of the following 3 stitches, sc 2 into the next stitch (1 increase)* rep from *to* another 5 times (30 stitches).
RND 6: sc 1, *sc 2 into the next stitch (1 increase), sc 1 into each of the following 4 stitches*, rep from *to* another 5 times (36 stitches).
Sl st 1 to close round, cut yarn and fasten off.

Large element b

With the lobster red follow the instructions given for the medium element b, at the end of round 6 do not cut yarn but proceed as follows:
RND 7 : *sc 1 into each of the following 5 stitches, sc 2 into the next stitch (1 increase)* rep from *to* another 5 times (42 stitches).

RND 8: sc 1 into each of the following 2 stitches, *sc 2 into the next stitch (1 increase), sc 1 into each of the following 4 stitches*, rep from *to* another 5 times (48 stitches). Sl st 1 to close round, cut yarn and fasten off.

With the orange yarn insert hook into any one of the stitches forming the last round of the round disk elements, ch 1 to fasten on yarn, then *sl st 1 and ch1 in next stitch*; rep from *to* to the end of the round, ss 1 to close round. Cut and fasten off yarn.
Rep on all three elements.

Position the three round elements on top of one another as shown and stitch them together on reverse with neat, invisible stitches, then sew the decoration into position onto the hair band.

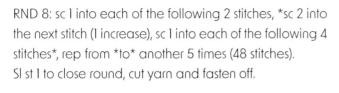

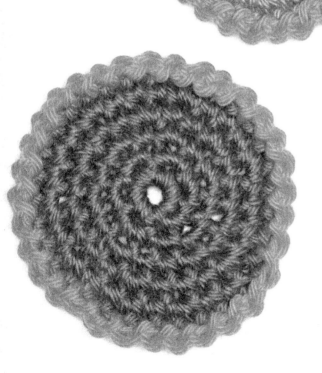

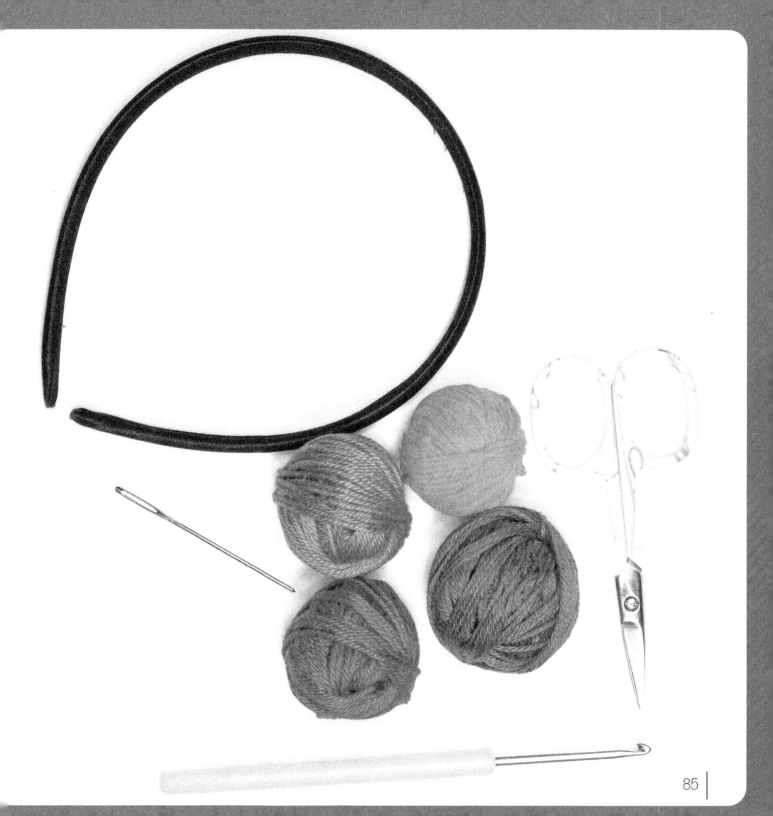

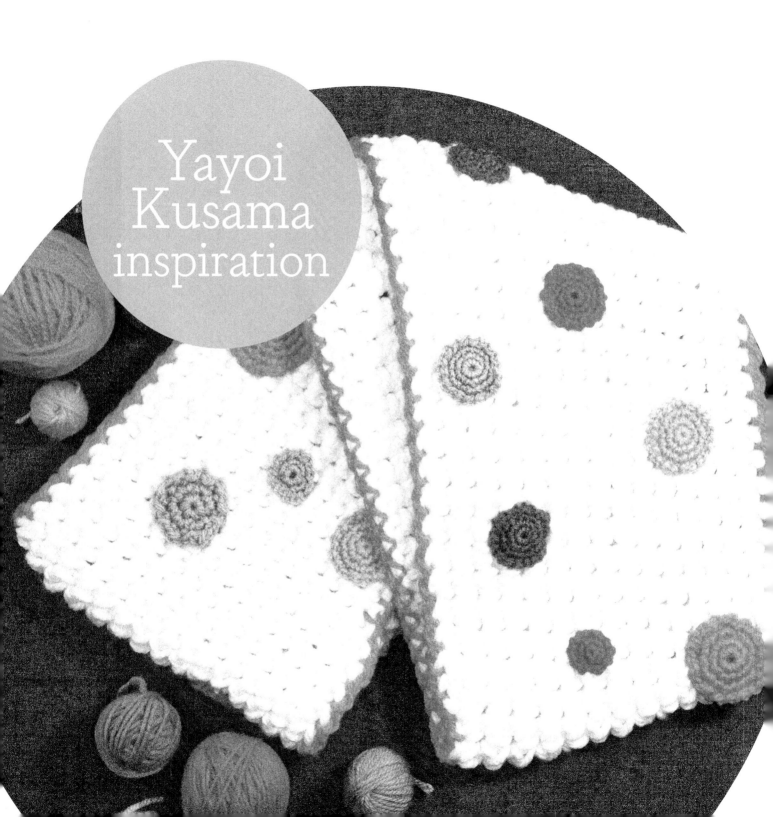

Yayoi
Kusama
inspiration

Polka Dot Warmer

I made this warmer as a tribute to Polka Dots Power and to the artist Yoyo Kusama.

MATERIALS

100% acrylic | super bulky (6) weight yarn (7oz = 131yds / 200g = 120m) | color:cream
crochet hook size N/P-15 (10 mm)
100% acrylic | bulky (5) weight yarn (3.5oz = 180yds / 100g = 165m) | color:orange
yarn needle
a lot of polka dots in assorted sizes and colors pink, red, orange, dark green, light green

PATTERN STITCHES

ch, sl st, sc

INSTRUCTIONS

Follow the instructions given for the Snood. Make the trimming following the instructions for the Fitted Neck Warmer using the orange color yarn. Add the same finishing border on polka dots. Sew the polka dots in random order.

LET ME SHOW YOU

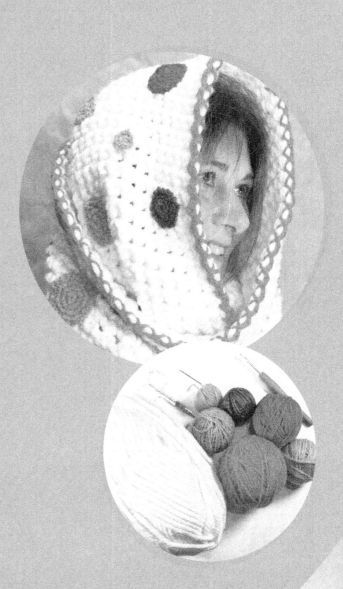

Ring
Dreamcatcher

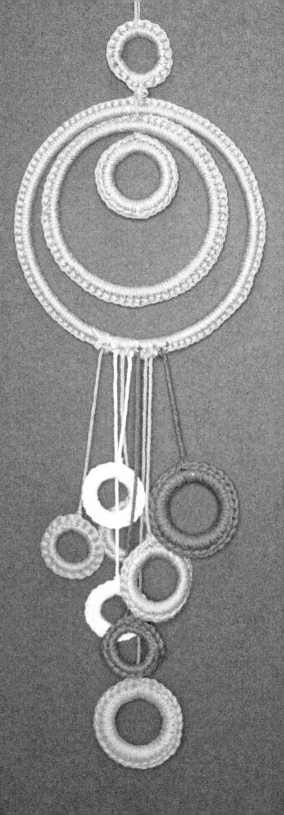

Ring Dreamcatcher

MATERIALS

100% cotton | fine (2) weight yarn (1.75oz = 137yds / 50g = 125m)

about 1oz (30 g) is required in each of the following colors: bright green, red, light yellow, lobster red

crochet hook C-2 or D-3 (3.25 – 3.75 mm)

yarn needle

no. 3 large plastic rings, size 1.57" (4 cm)

no. 2 medium plastic rings, size 1.18" (3 cm)

no. 6 small plastic rings, size 0.98" (2.5 cm)

no. 1 metal ring (ring A), size 4" (10 cm)

no. 1 metal ring (ring B), size 2.8" (7 cm)

PATTERN STITCHES

ch, sl st, sc

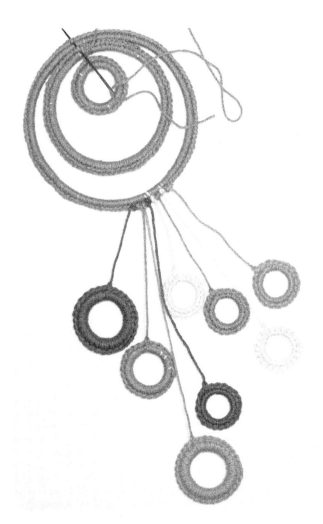

LET ME SHOW YOU

Materials

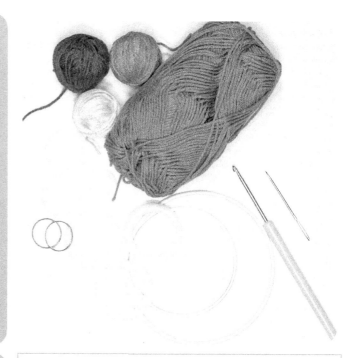

Step-by-step instructions

Using the red, light yellow, light orange, lobster red and green yarn, sc over all the large, medium and small plastic rings (as instructed in steps 1 to 7 at pages 16 and 17), each one in a different color.

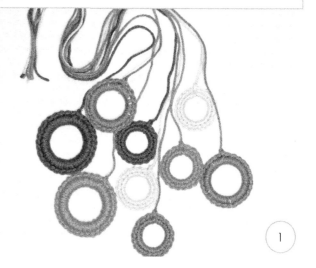

1

With the green yarn, sc over the 2 metal rings (A and B). Cut and fasten off ends.

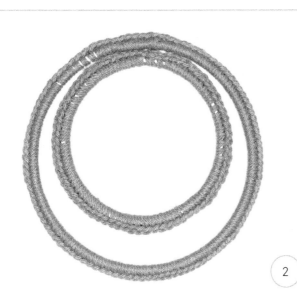

(2)

Attach the small rings to the larger ring (A) in random order (fasten each one with a triple knot).

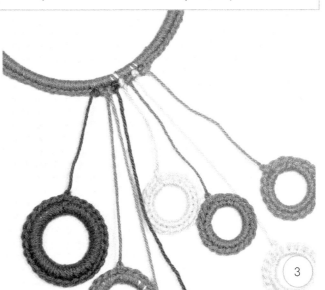

(3)

Sew together ring A, ring B ring and the last large ring done in green.

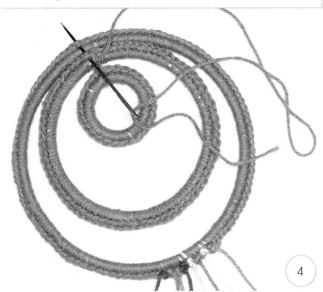

(4)

Sew on the last small ring done in green.

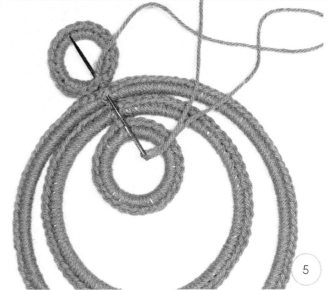

(5)

Hanging Ring Mobile

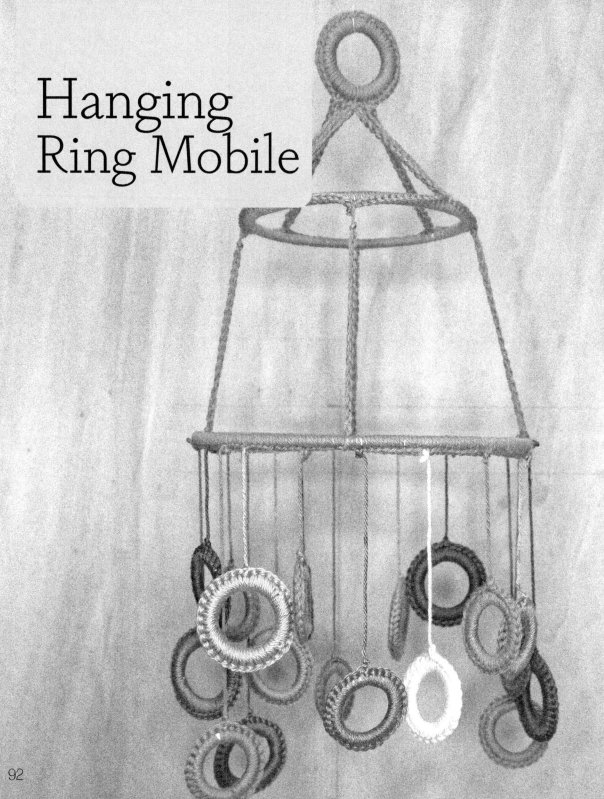

Hanging Ring Mobile

MATERIALS

100% cotton | fine (2) weight yarn (1.75oz = 137yds / 50g = 125m)

about 1.75 oz (50 g) is required in each of the following colors: bright green, pink, light pink, wisteria violet, cyclamen purple

crochet hook C-2 or D-3 (3.25 – 3.75 mm)

yarn needle

4 stitch markers

no. 9 large plastic rings, size 1.57" (4 cm)

no. 10 medium plastic rings, size 1.18" (3 cm)

no. 8 small plastic rings, size 0.98" (2.5 cm)

no. 1 metal ring (ring A), size 6" (15 cm)

no. 1 metal ring (ring B), size 4" (10 cm)

PATTERN STITCHES

ch, sl st, sc

LET ME SHOW YOU

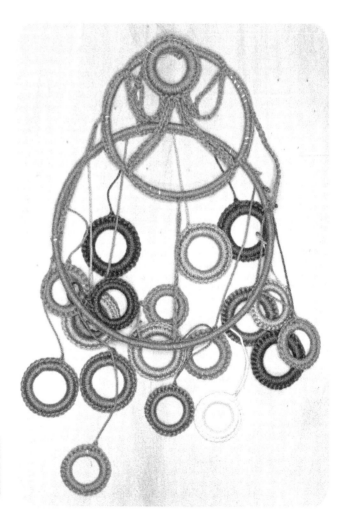

Step-by-step instructions

With the green yarn, sc over the 2 metal rings (A and B). Cut and fasten off yarn.

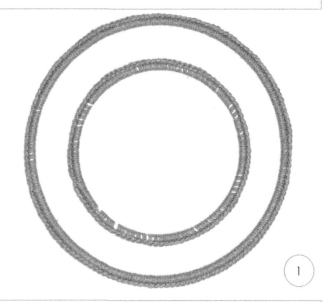

(1)

Attach the small rings to ring (A) in random colored order ensuring that they are spaced out at regular intervals from one another.

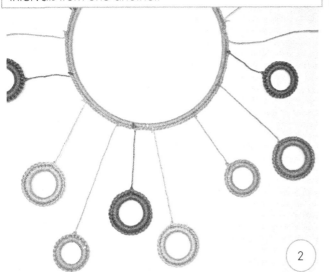

(2)

Using a stitch marker, mark out 4 stitches located at regular intervals from one another on the B ring (i.e. mark out the 4 quarter points).

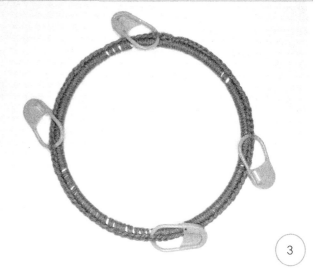

(3)

Using the pink, light pink, wisteria violet, cyclamen purple and green yarn, cover all the plastic rings (as instructed in steps 1 to 7 at pages 16 and 17).
Remember to set one of the small plastic rings aside for use in step 5.

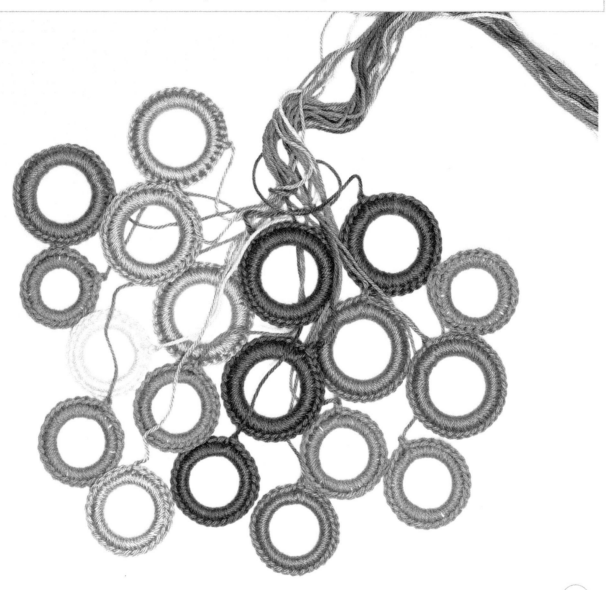

with the green yarn, single crochet around the small plastic ring previously set aside, sl st 1 into the first sc of the round. Do not cut yarn.
ch 15, insert hook into one of the 4 marked stitches on the green B ring, remove stitch marker and sl st 1 to join on yarn, then ch 15, sl st 1 back into the small ring, skipping about a quarter of the stitches done to cover it*.

rep from *to* another 3 times, cut and fasten off yarn, working in all ends.

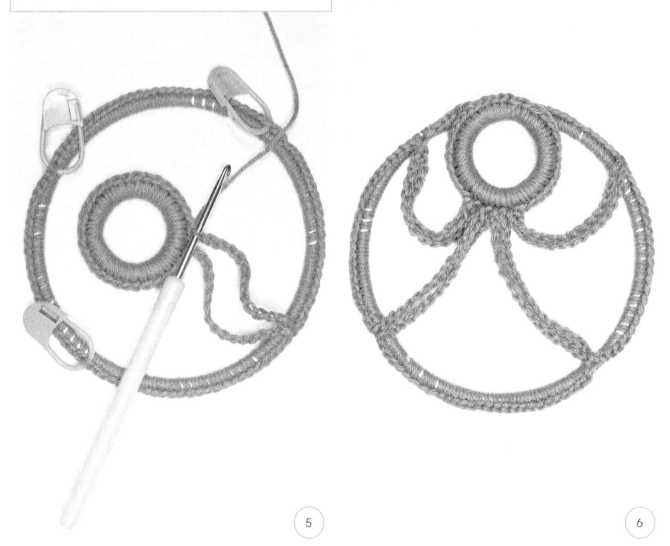

5

6

with the green yarn, crochet a total of 6 chains 6"(15 cm) long and use them to connect the two green rings (A and B) to one another, fastening each tail end with a triple knot.

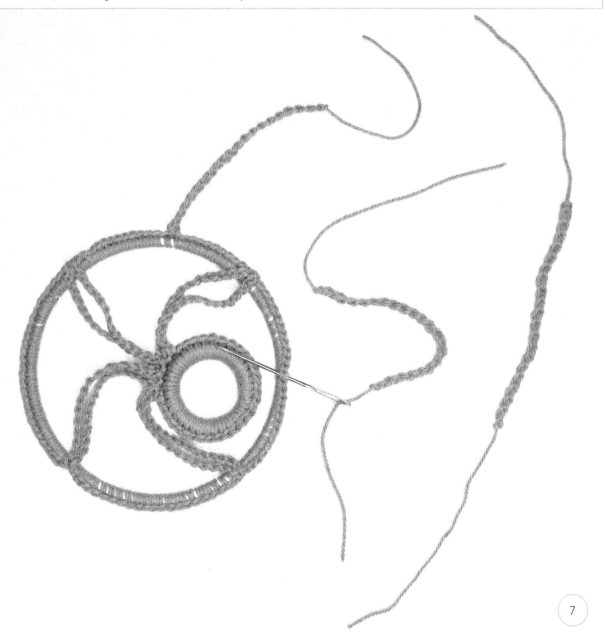

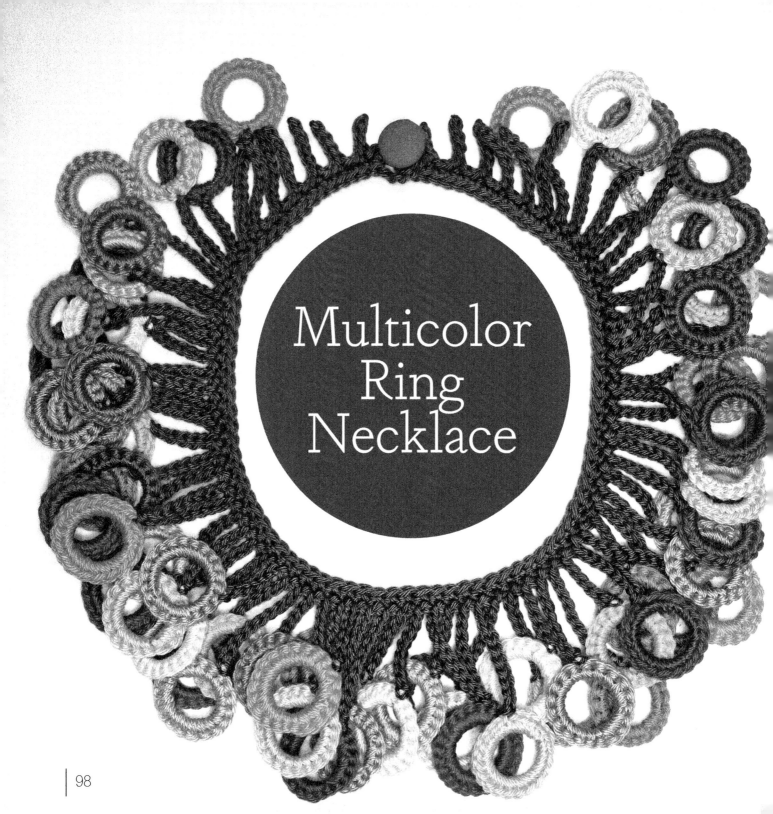

Multicolor
Ring
Necklace

Multicolor Ring Necklace

MATERIALS

100% cotton | fine (2) weight yarn (1.75oz = 137yds / 50g = 125m)

1.75 oz (50 g) color: dark green, plus

about 1.75 oz (50 g) is required in each of the following colors: bright green, lobster red, light pink, violet, cyclamen purple, light blue, royal blue, orange, turquoise, burgundy and purple

crochet hook C-2 or D-3 (3.25 b 3.75 mm)

yarn needle

no. 70 small 1" (2.5 cm) diameter plastic or metal rings (or number of rings to your liking, depending on length of necklace)

1 button having a max diameter of about 2/3 of an inch (1.5 cm)

PATTERN STITCHES

ch, sl st, sc

decorative fringe stitch: ch4(5,6,7,8,10) insert hook into 2nd chain from hook, sl st 1 into each chain back across, sl st 1 back into the stitch you started out from

LET ME SHOW YOU

Materials

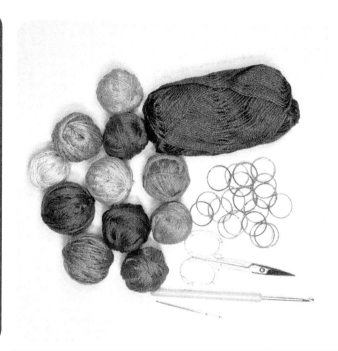

Step-by-step instructions

Using bright green, lobster red, light pink, wisteria violet, cyclamen purple, light blue, royal blue, orange, turquoise, burgundy, violet yarn, cover all the plastic rings in single crochet (as instructed in steps 1 to 7 at pages 16 and 17). Cut and fasten off yarn.

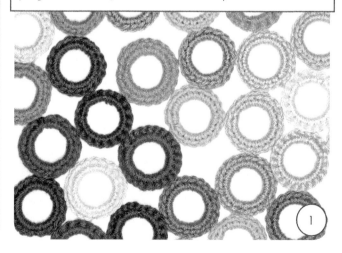

With the dark green make a chain long enough to fit you. For my necklace, I chained 91, i.e. approx. 19" (48 cm).

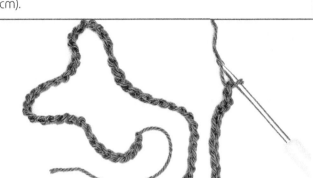

(2)

ROW 1: insert hook in the 2nd ch from hook

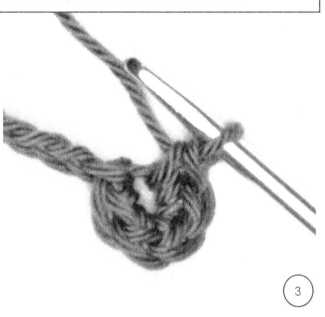

(3)

sc 1 into each of the following chains

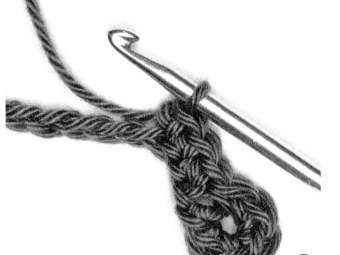

(4)

inserting hook in the back loop only of each chain

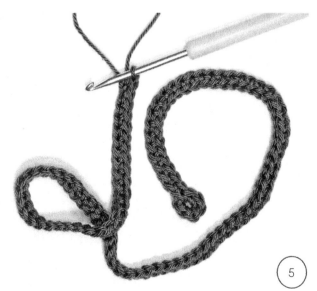

(5)

when at end of row, make a chain for the eyelet (for my necklace, I chained 10)

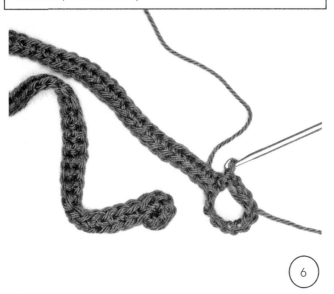

(6)

slst 1 back into the first chain to close eyelet ring,

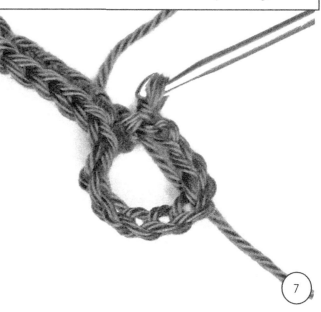

(7)

cut yarn and fasten off yarn tail on back of work

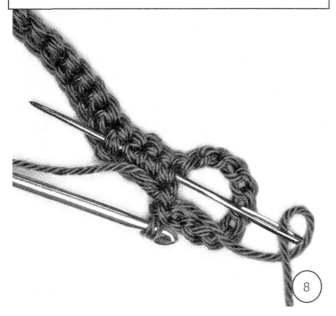

(8)

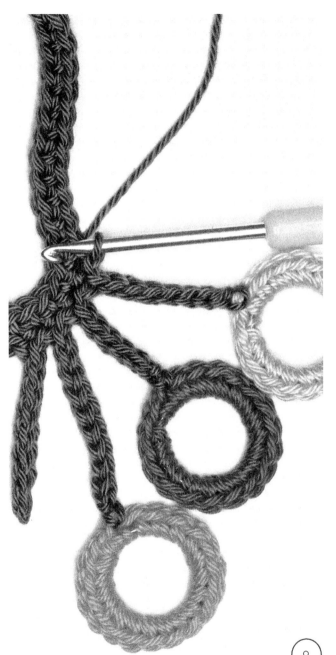

ROW 2: in first 15 stitches of row: sl st 1, then make 1 ch 4 fringe stitch, sl st 1 into next stitch, 1 ch 5 fringe stitch, sl st 1 into next stitch, 1 ch 6 fringe stitch, sl st 1 into next stitch, 1 ch 7 fringe stitch, sl st 1 into next stitch, 1 ch 8 fringe stitch, sl st 1 into next stitch, 1 ch 9 fringe stitch sl st 1 into next stitch, 1 ch 10 fringe stitch, sl st 1 into next stitch.

In following stitches make *1 ch 6 fringe stitch, sl st 1 into next stitch, 1 ch 7 fringe stitch, sl st 1 into next stitch, 1 ch 8 fringe stitch, sl st 1 into next stitch, 1 ch 9 fringe stitch sl st 1 into next stitch, 1 ch 10 fringe stitch, sl st 1 into next stitch, 1 ch 9 fringe stitch, sl st 1 into next stitch, 1 ch 8 fringe stitch, sl st 1 into next stitch, 1 ch 7 fringe stitch, sl st 1 into next stitch, 1 ch 6 fringe stitch sl st 1 into next stitch*, rep *to* sequence until you have 14 stitches left in your row.

N.B.:
- as you make the fringe stitches from * to *, attach all the rings in random colored order and evenly spaced as illustrated and as instructed in steps 10 to 12 at pages 38 and 39.
- it doesn't matter if you do not finish a sequence, as that depends on the number of chains you started out with.

In last 14 stitches of row: make 1 ch 10 fringe stitch, sl st 1 into next stitch, 1 ch 9 fringe stitch, sl st 1 into next stitch, 1 ch 8 fringe stitch, sl st 1 into next stitch, 1 ch 7 fringe stitch, sl st 1 into next stitch, 1 ch 6 fringe stitch, sl st 1 into next stitch, 1 ch 5 fringe stitch sl st 1 into next stitch, 1 ch 4 fringe stitch, sl st 1 into last stitch. Cut and fasten off yarn.

(9)

decorative fringe stitch with ring attached: after making the fringe stitch chain in given length, remove hook from yarn loop, insert hook into both loops of one of the single crochet stitches worked around the selected ring, insert hook back into the yarn loop,

pull the yarn loop through the single crochet stitch so that ring is attached,

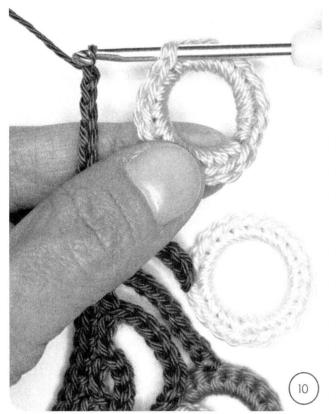

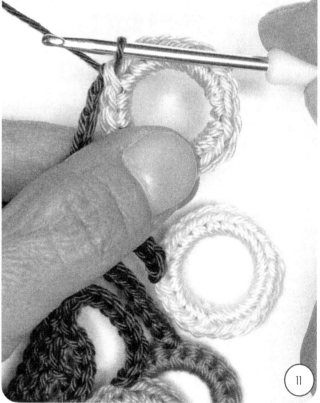

then sl st 1 into each chain back across.
Rep step 10 to step 12 for all decorative fringe stitches with ring attached.
Sew button to end of row 1 as illustrated.

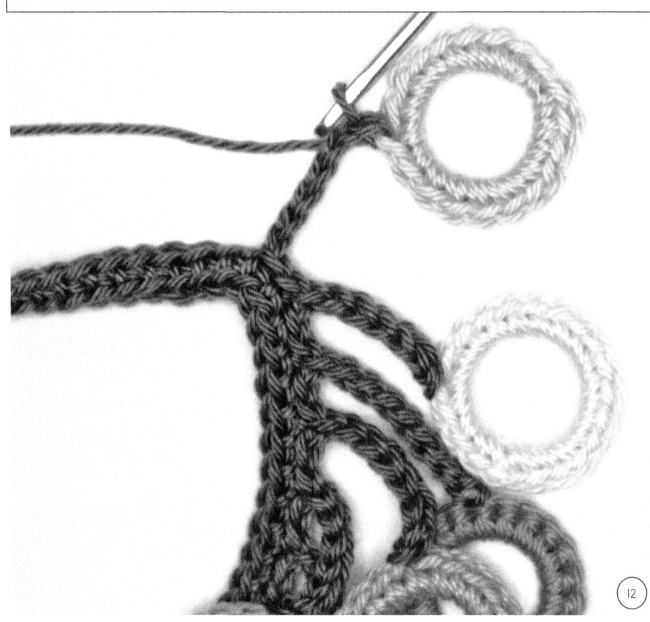

(12)

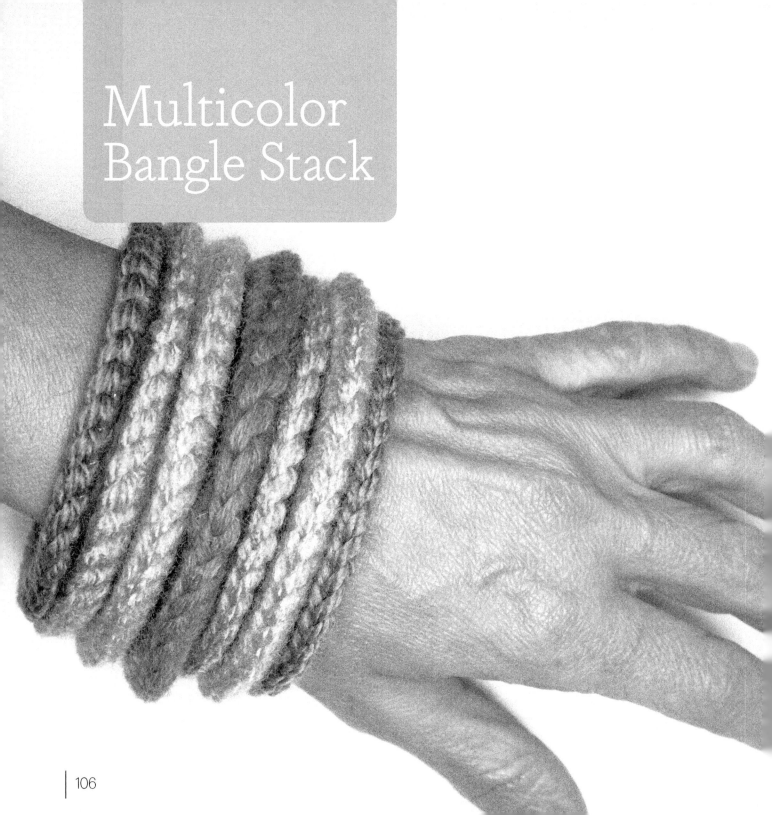

Multicolor Bangle Stack

Multicolor Bangle Stack

MATERIALS

100% acrylic | bulky (5) weight yarn (3.5oz = 180yds / 100g = 165m) | color: celadon green, light pink, wisteria violet, light yellow
crochet hook size I-9 (5.50 mm)
yarn needle
recycled metal (or plastic) bangles, any bangle you no longer use, to use as a base to crochet over

PATTERN STITCHES

ch, sl st, sc

INSTRUCTIONS

Using the celadon green, light pink, wisteria violet and light yellow yarn, single crochet over each bangle following the instructions given in steps 1 to 7 at pages 16 and 17.
Cut and fasten off yarn.

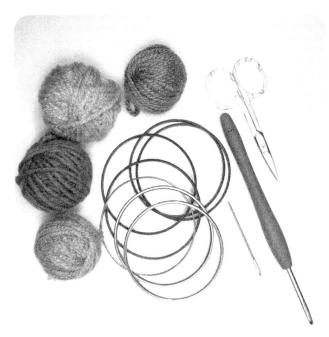

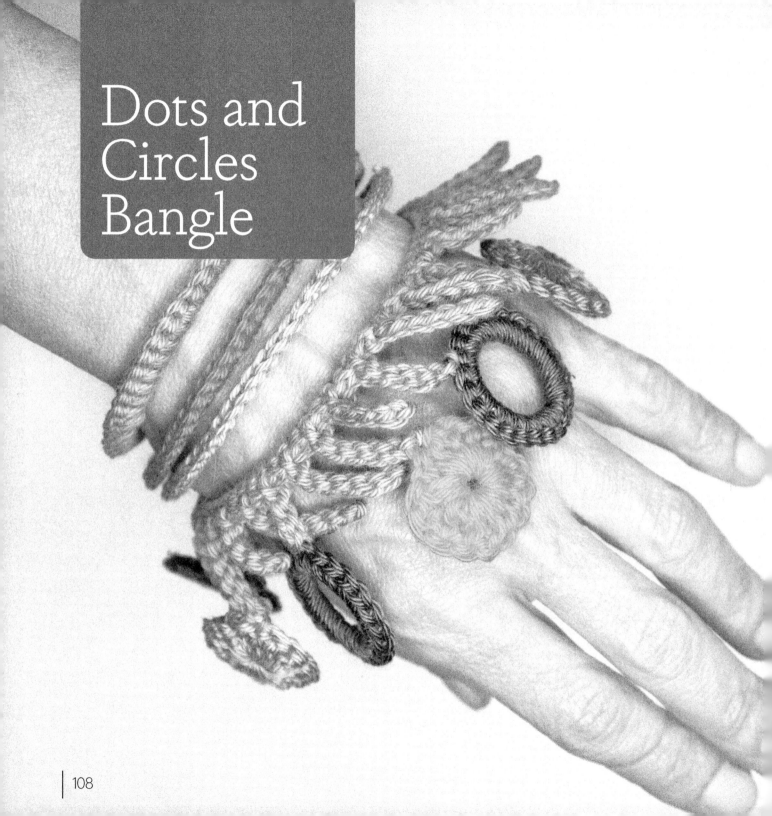

Dots and Circles Bangle

Dots and Circles Bangle

MATERIALS

100% cotton | fine (2) weight yarn (1.75oz = 137yds / 50g = 125m)

about 0,5oz (15 g) is required in each of the following colors: bright green, dark green, orange, light yellow, light pink, light blue,

cyclamen purple, burgundy, turquoise

crochet hook C-2 or D-3 (3.25 – 3.75 mm)

yarn needle

no. 4 recycled metal (or plastic) bangles

no. 5 small metal (or plastic) rings, size 0.98" (2.5 cm)

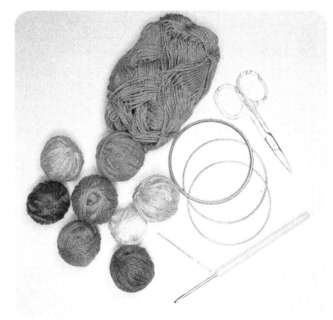

PATTERN STITCHES

ch, sl st, sc

Decorative fringe stitch: ch 5(6,8,10), insert hook into 2nd ch from hook and sl st 1 into each of the following ch)

LET ME SHOW YOU

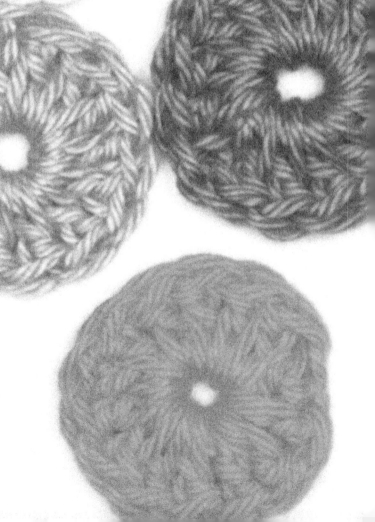

Step 1
Decorative disc shaped elements

(make each one in a different color in orange, light yellow, light blue, cyclamen purple, burgundy, turquoise)

ch 5 and join to form a circle.

RND 1: make a a number of dc sufficient enough to cover the chain circle completely (approx. dc 15).

Cut and fasten off thread.

Decorative rings

Decorative rings

(make 5)

Using the dark green yarn sc around all the small metal rings (as instructed in steps 1 to 7 at pages 16 and 17).

Cut and fasten off thread.

Using the turquoise, orange and bright green yarn, cover 3 of the metal bangles in the same manner. Set the 4th bangle aside.

Cut and fasten off yarn.

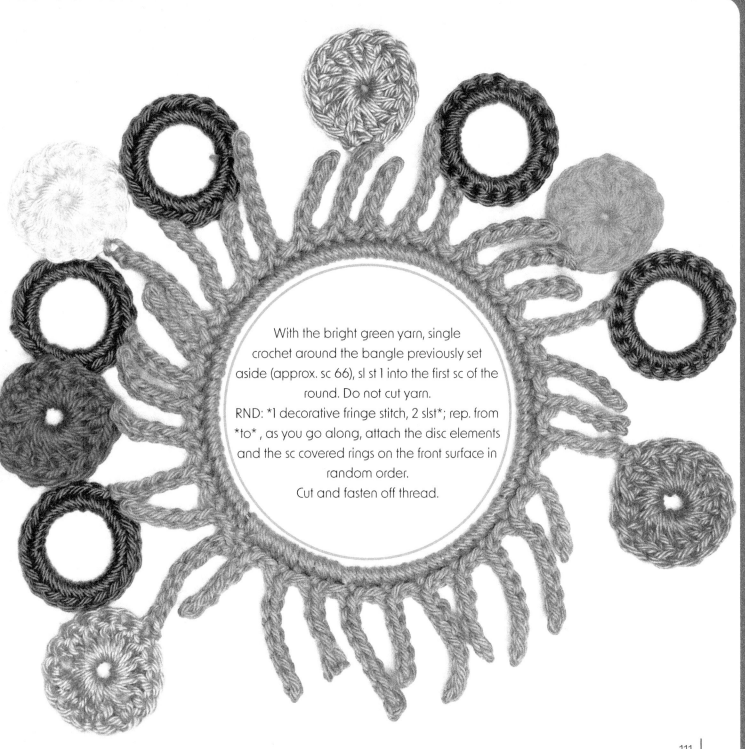

With the bright green yarn, single crochet around the bangle previously set aside (approx. sc 66), sl st 1 into the first sc of the round. Do not cut yarn.

RND: *1 decorative fringe stitch, 2 slst*; rep. from *to* , as you go along, attach the disc elements and the sc covered rings on the front surface in random order.

Cut and fasten off thread.

Multicolor
Beaded
Ring

Multicolor Beaded Ring

MATERIALS

SUPER FINE (1) weight (1.75 oz = 213 yards /50 g = 195 m) 100% high quality mercerized cotton thread:

about half an oz (± 15 g) is required in a lilac shade

steel hook size 8 (1.50 mm) or size 8/4 (1.25 mm), depending on your individual crocheting tension

yarn needle

fiber- fill or toy stuffing

1 metal ring blank with a tray bezel to fit the size of your crochet bead

assorted plastic beads

Select shape, style, color, wire thickness and material of metal findings to your liking.

PATTERN STITCHES

ch, sl st, sc

PATTERN NOTES

The ring is composed of one crochet bead made up of 2 sections worked separately (front and rear) in continuous crochet rounds. The sections are then joined together in the course of the project, the crochet bead is attached to the bezel and decorated with plastic beads.

INSTRUCTIONS
FOR THE CROCHET BEAD
SECTION 1 (REAR)

with the lilac thread form a double loop and insert hook,

RND 1: ch 1, sc 6.

RND 2: *sc 2 in each stitch*, rep from *to* another 5 times (12 stitches).

RND 3: *sc 1, sc 2 in the following stitch (1 increase)*; rep from *to* another 5 times (18 stitches).

RND 4: *sc 2 in next stitch (1 increase), sc 1 in following 2 stitches*; rep from *to* another 5 times (24 stitches), sl st 1 to close round. Cut and fasten off thread.

SECTION 2 (FRONT)

Follow the instructions given for section 1 here above, but do not cut thread and fasten off after round 4.

RND 5, 6, 7: sc 1 into each stitch around. Do not cut thread and fasten off after round 7.

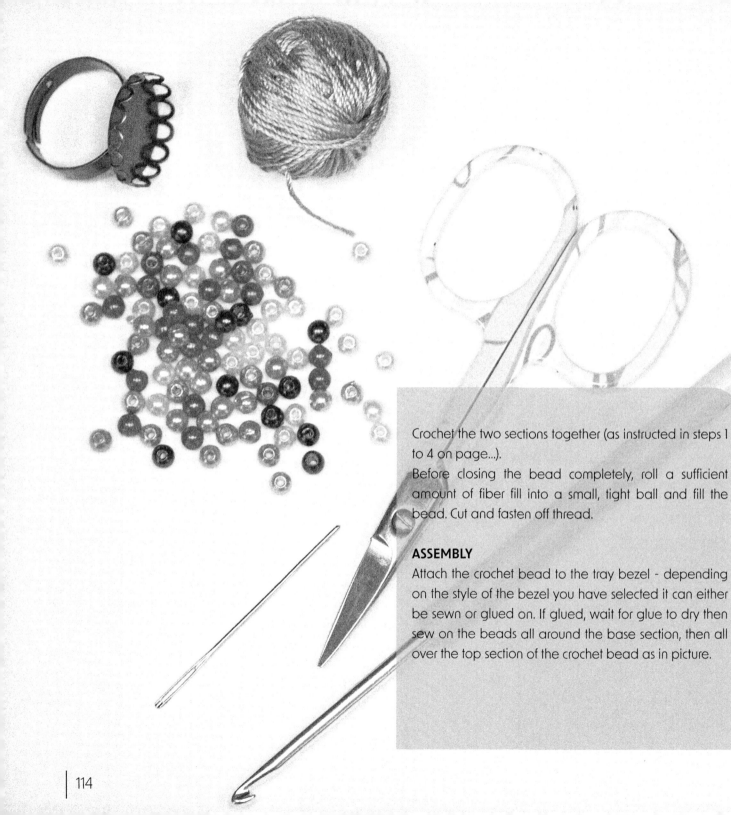

Crochet the two sections together (as instructed in steps 1 to 4 on page...).

Before closing the bead completely, roll a sufficient amount of fiber fill into a small, tight ball and fill the bead. Cut and fasten off thread.

ASSEMBLY

Attach the crochet bead to the tray bezel - depending on the style of the bezel you have selected it can either be sewn or glued on. If glued, wait for glue to dry then sew on the beads all around the base section, then all over the top section of the crochet bead as in picture.

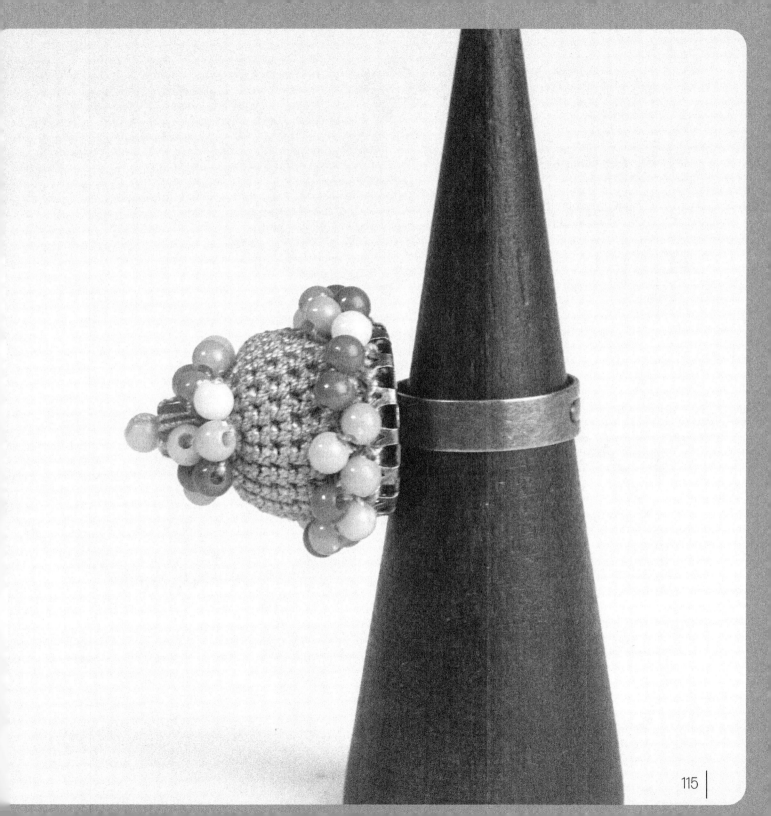

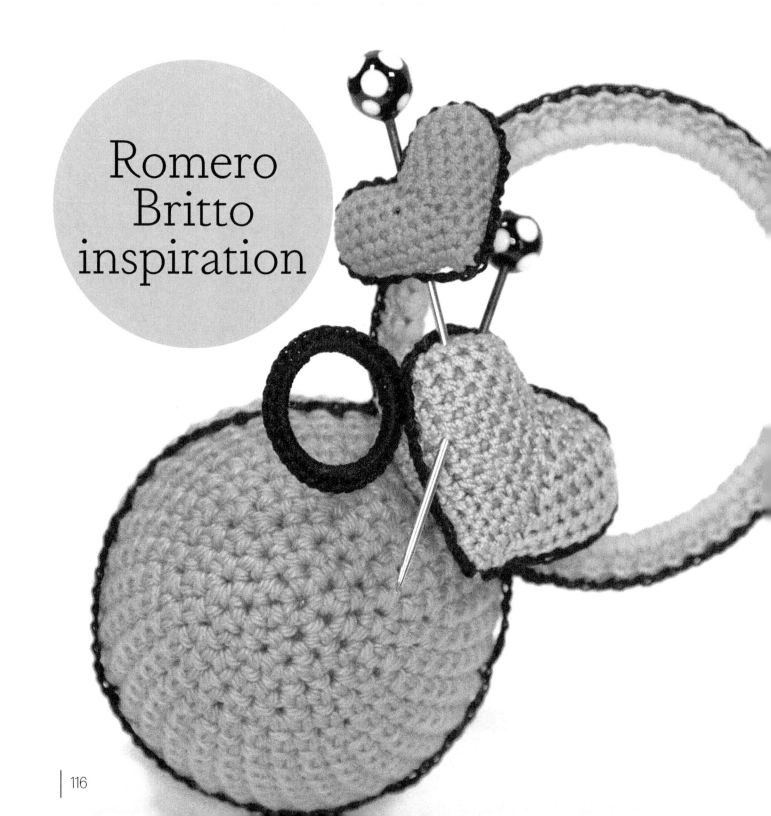

Romero
Britto
inspiration

Soft Sculpture inspired by Romero Britto

I designed this soft sculpture as a tribute to the power of heart shapes and to Romero Britto, the famous Brazilian artist.

MATERIALS

SUPER FINE (1) weight (1.75 oz = 191 yards /50 g = 175 m) 100% high quality mercerized cotton thread: about half an oz (± 15 g) colors: red, mustard yellow, black, fuchsia steel hook size 4/0 (1.75 mm) or size 8 (1.50 mm), depending on your individual crocheting tension yarn needle

100% cotton | fine (2) weight yarn (1.75oz = 137yds / 50g = 125m) about 0,5oz (15 g) colors: fuchsia, orange crochet hook C-2 or D-3 (3.25 – 3.75 mm) yarn needle

no. 1 plastic ball having a diameter of 3" (8 cm) fiber-fill or toy stuffing no. 1 recycled metal (or plastic) bangle no. 1 small metal (or plastic) ring, size 0.98" (2.5 cm) no. 2 hatpins

PATTERN STITCHES

ch, sl st, sc

LET ME SHOW YOU

The soft sculpture is composed of 5 crochet elements: 1 fuchsia crochet ball, 1 small red heart, 1 medium mustard yellow heart and 2 crocheted rings. The composition is then embellished with 2 hatpins.

INSTRUCTIONS
RED HEART

For the first cup section, with the red SUPER FINE yarn, form a double loop and insert hook

RND 1: ch 1, sc 6.

RND 2: *sc 2 in each stitch*, rep from *to* another 5 times (12 stitches).

RND 3, 4, 5: sc 1 into each stitch around. Sl st 1 to close round, cut yarn and fasten off.

For the second cup section, follow the same instructions given for the first but do not cut yarn after round 5, so that you have one loop left on your hook.

To join the two cup sections together, place them one alongside the other as illustrated on page....:

With the inside of cup section 2 facing you and your one loop already on hook, insert hook simultaneously through the next stitch in cup section 2 and a corresponding sc stitch in cup section 1, then sc 1.

Make another 2 sc in the same manner over the next 2 stitches. This forms a neat central seam that firmly holds the two cup sections together.

With the inside of cup section 2 facing you continue making sc 1 into each of the next 8 stitches

Insert hook into the last stitch of cup section 2, yarn over and draw up a loop, insert hook into the first stitch of cup section 1, yarn over and draw up a loop:

you now have 3 loops on your hook, yarn over and draw through all 3 loops on hook (1 decrease)

sc 1 into the next 7 stitches around, decrease 1.

sc 1 into the next 6 stitches around, insert hook into the following stitch, yarn over and draw up a loop, insert hook into the following stitch, yarn over and draw up a loop, insert hook into the following stitch, yarn over and draw up a loop: you now have 4 loops on your hook yarn over and draw through all 4 loops on hook (2 decreases)

sc 1 into the next 5 stitches around, decrease 2

Proceed crocheting in spiral rounds, always working in 2 decreases on top of the decreases made in the previous round. Cut and fasten off thread.

MUSTARD YELLOW HEART

For the first cup section, with the mustard yellow SUPER FINE yarn, follow the instructions given for the red heart, RND 1 and 2

RND 3: *sc 1, sc 2 in the following stitch (1 increase)*; rep from *to* another 5 times (18 stitches).

RND 4: *sc 2 in next stitch (1 increase), sc 1 in following 2 stitches*; rep from *to* another 5 times (24 stitches).

RND 5, 6, 7, 8: sc 1 into each stitch around. Sl st 1 to close round, cut yarn and fasten off.

For the second cup section, follow the same instructions given for the first but do not cut yarn after round 8, so that you have one loop left on your hook.

To join the two cup sections together, place them one alongside the other as illustrated on page....:

With the inside of cup section 2 facing you and your one loop already on hook, insert hook simultaneously through the next stitch in cup section 2 and a corresponding sc stitch in cup section 1, then sc 1.

Make another 4 sc in the same manner over the next 4 stitches. This forms a neat central seam that firmly holds the two cup sections together.

With the inside of cup section 2 facing you continue making sc 1 into each of the next 18 stitches
decrease 1, sc 1 into the next 17 stitches around, decrease 1
sc 1 into the next 16 stitches around,
decrease 2, sc 1 into the next 15 stitches around, decrease 2
Proceed crocheting in spiral rounds, always working in 2 decreases on top of the decreases made in the previous round.
Cut and fasten off thread.

ORANGE RING

Using the orange yarn, sc crochet to cover the metal bangle
Cut and fasten off yarn.
With the SUPER FINE fuchsia yarn insert hook into any one of the stitches along the row, ch 1 to fasten on yarn. Then *sl st 1 and ch1 in next stitch*; rep
from *to* to the end of the round, ss 1 to close round. Cut and fasten off yarn.
With the SUPER FINE black yarn insert hook into the back loop of any one of the stitches along the row, ch 1 to fasten on yarn. sl st to the end of the round.
Cut and fasten off yarn.

BLACK RING

With the SUPER FINE black yarn, sc crochet to cover the small metal ring.
Cut and fasten off yarn.

FUCHSIA CROCHET BALL

This ball is made up starting with two half circle sections that are crocheted separately and then joined together.

Follow the step by step instructions in "Crochet for beginners" Vol.1 QRCODE

HALF CIRCLE SECTION 1

WIth the cotton fine (2) fuchsia yarn for the section1 form a double loop and insert hook
RND 1: ch 1, sc 6.
RND 2: *sc 2 in each stitch*, rep from *to* another 5 times (12 stitches).
RND 3: *sc 1, sc 2 in the following stitch (1 increase)*; rep from *to* another 5 times (18 stitches).
RND 4: *sc 2 in next stitch (1 increase), sc 1 in following 2 stitches*; rep from *to* another 5 times (24 stitches).
RND 5: *sc 1 into each of the following 3 stitches, sc 2 into the next stitch (1 increase)* rep from *to* another 5 times (30 stitches).
RND 6, 7, 8, 9, 10: sc 1 into each stitch around, sl st 1 to close last round. Cut yarn and fasten off.

HALF CIRCLE SECTION 2

Follow the same instructions given for section 1, cut and fasten off the yarn leaving an end approx.
10 inches (25 cm) long for sewing the two half circle sections together. Remembering in good time to insert the plastic ball (or to gradually stuff with fiber-fill). Fasten off and work in tail end.

ASSEMBLY

With the black make a row of chain stitches long enough for sewing onto the crochet hearts, ball and rings.
Sew the crochet elements together with tight, neat invisible stitches as shown in the picture.
Decorate with the two hatpins.

Dangle
Earrings

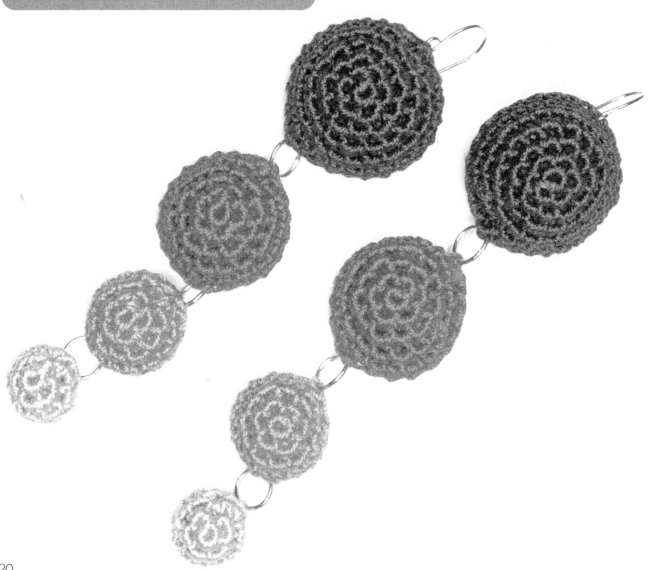

Dangle Earrings

MATERIALS

SUPER FINE (1) weight (1.75 oz = 191 yards /50 g = 175 m) 100% high quality mercerized cotton thread: about half an oz (± 15 g) is required in each of the following colors: burgundy, red, pink, light pink

steel hook size 4/0 (1.75 mm) or size 8 (1.50 mm), depending on your individual crocheting tension

yarn needle

fiber- fill or toy stuffing

no. 2 metal earring wires

no. 6 or 8 metal open jump rings, round, with a 6 mm outer diameter

flat nosed jewelry pliers

Select shape, style, color, wire thickness and material of metal findings to your liking.

PATTERN STITCHES

ch, sl st, sc

PATTERN NOTES

Each earring is composed of 4 crochet elements (crochet beads).

All the crochet beads are made up of 2 sections worked separately (front and rear) in continuous crochet rounds. The sections are then join together in the course of the project.

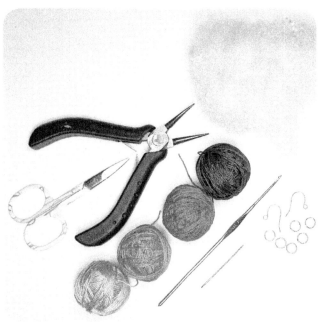

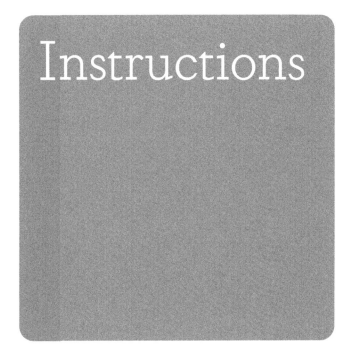

Instructions

LIGHT PINK CROCHET BEAD (MAKE 2!)

Section 1 (rear)

With the light pink, form a double loop and insert hook
RND 1: ch 1, sc 6.

RND 2: *sc 2 in each stitch*, rep from *to* another 5 times (12 stitches), sl st 1 to close round. Cut and fasten off thread.

Section 2 (front)

Follow the instructions given for section 1 here above but do not cut thread and fasten off after round 2.

Crochet the two sections together (as instructed in Steps 1 to 4 on page...).

Before closing the bead completely, roll a sufficient amount of fiber fill into a small, tight ball and fill the bead. Cut and fasten off thread.

PINK CROCHET BEADS (MAKE 2!)

Section 1 (rear)

With the pink, follow the instructions given for section 1 of the light pink crochet beads, but do not cut thread and fasten off after round 2.

RND 3: *sc 1, sc 2 in the following stitch (1 increase)*; rep from *to* another 5 times (18 stitches), sl st 1 to close round. Cut and fasten off thread.

Section 2 (front)

Follow the instructions given for section 1 here above, but do not cut thread and fasten off after round 3.

Crochet the two sections together (as instructed in Steps 1 to 4 on page...).

Before closing the bead completely, roll a sufficient amount of fiber fill into a small, tight ball and fill the bead. Cut and fasten off thread.

RED CROCHET BEADS (MAKE 2!)
Section 1 (rear)
With the red follow the instructions given for section 1 of the pink crochet beads, but do not cut thread and fasten off after round 3.

RND 4: *sc 2 in next stitch (1 increase), sc 1 in following 2 stitches*; rep from *to* another 5 times (24 stitches), sl st 1 to close round. Cut and fasten off thread.

Section 2 (front)
Follow the instructions given for section 1 here above, but do not cut thread and fasten off after round 4.

Crochet the two sections together (as instructed in Steps 1 to 4 on page...).

Before closing the bead completely, roll a sufficient amount of fiber fill into a small, tight ball and fill the bead. Cut and fasten off thread.

BURGUNDY CROCHET BEADS (MAKE 2!)
Section 1 (rear)
With the burgundy follow the instructions given for section 1 of the red crochet beads, but do not cut thread and fasten off after round 4.

RND 5: *sc 1 into each of the following 3 stitches, sc 2 into the next stitch (1 increase)* rep from *to* another 5 times (30 stitches), sl st 1 to close round. Cut and fasten off thread.

Section 2 (front)
Follow the instructions given for section 1 here above, but do not cut thread and fasten off after round 5.

Crochet the two sections together (as instructed in Steps 1 to 4 on page...).

Before closing the bead completely, roll a sufficient amount of fiber fill into a small, tight ball and fill the bead. Cut and fasten off thread.

ASSEMBLY
Using the open jump rings and the jewelry pliers, join the 4 beads belonging to each earring and attach the earring finding as in picture.

Alternatively to fiber-fill or toy stuffing, you can also use small round decorative aquarium glass stones, small glass marbles, old glass beads or small pebbles as filling for your crochet beads.

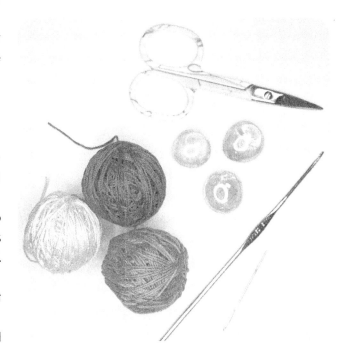

Sweet Little Flower

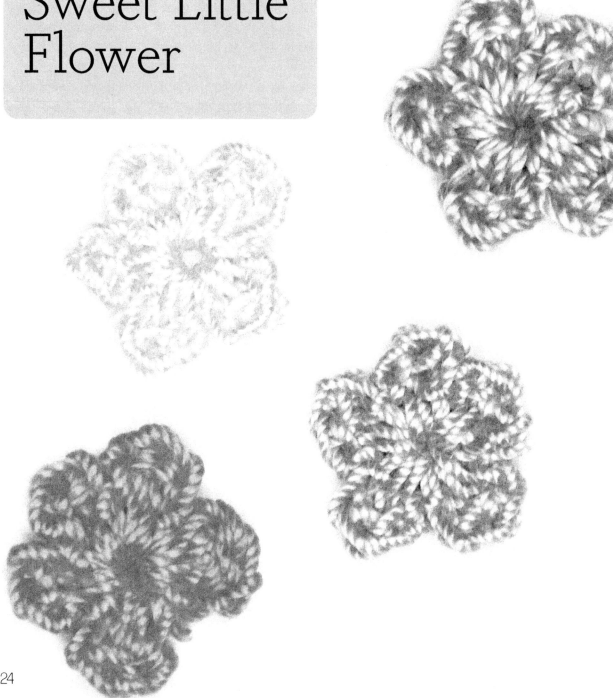

Sweet Little Flower

Of all the crochet appliques we can use to decorate and customize our creative projects, this five-petal crochet flower is certainly the easiest to make.

MATERIALS

Only a very small amount of yarn or thread is required to make this little flower so I suggest you use up all your leftover scraps and make a whole lot of them!
Use crochet hooks suitable to the yarn or thread weight you intend to use.

PATTERN STITCHES

ch, sl st, dc2tog

LET ME SHOW YOU

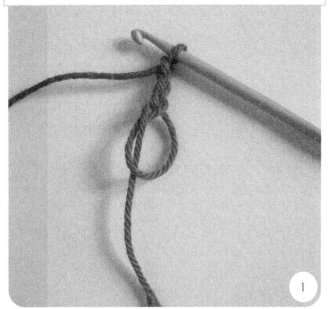

Step 1: form a double loop, *ch 3,

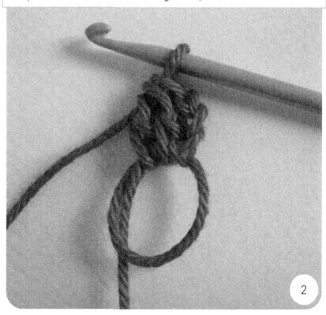

Step 2: double crochet 2 together,

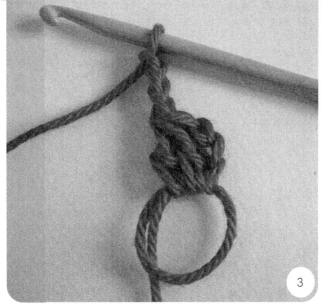

Step 3: ch 3,

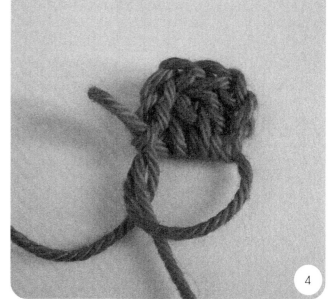

Step 4: sl st 1* (= first petal done)

Step 5: Following the above Steps *ch 3, dc2tog, ch 3, sl st 1*, make another 4 petals.

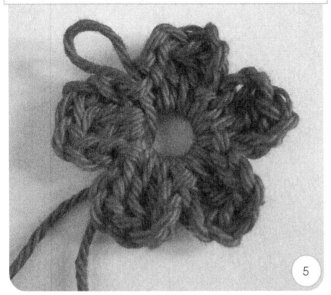

5

Step 6: Cut yarn and fasten off.

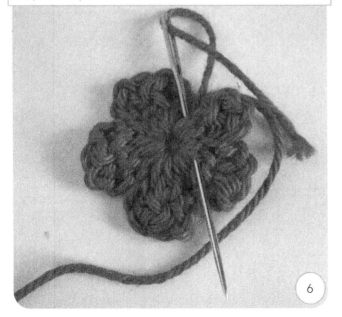

6

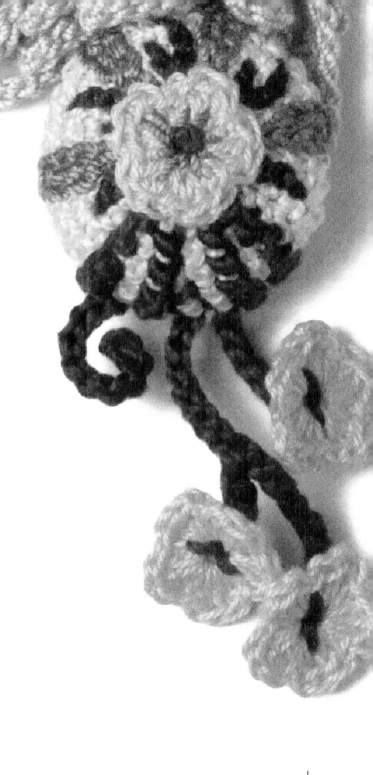

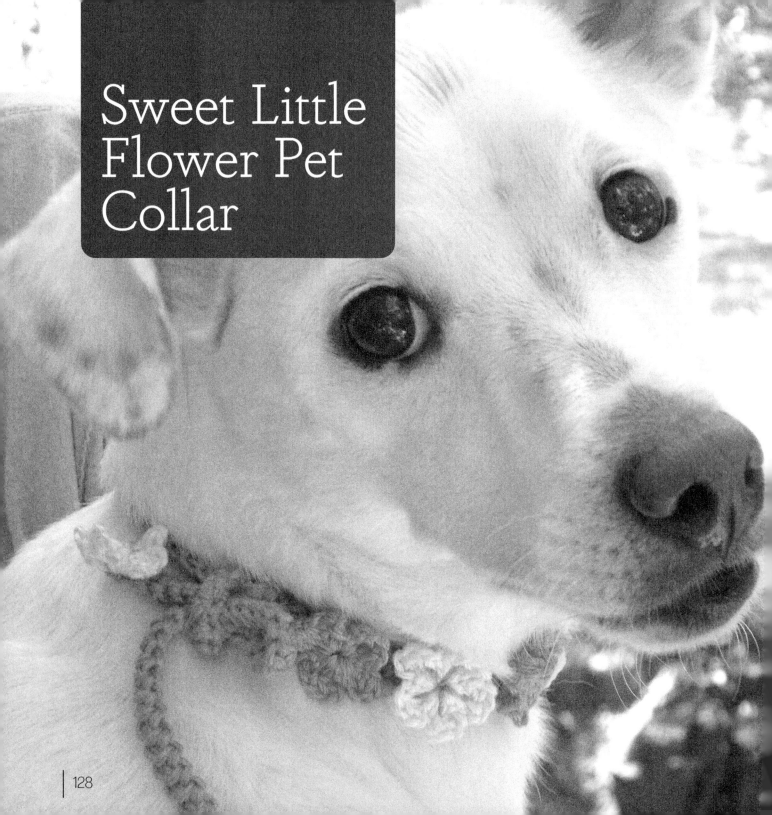

Sweet Little Flower Pet Collar

Sweet Little Flower Pet Collar

MATERIALS

100% cotton | fine (2) weight yarn (1.75oz = 137yds / 50g = 125m): about half an oz (15 g) in turquoise

an additional length (approx. 20") of 100% cotton crochet thread or embroidery floss in green

a total of 7 five-petal flowers (made as instructed in Steps 1 to 6 on pages 36-39) some in fuchsia and some in bright yellow

crochet hook sizes from a C-2 to a D-3 (2.75 to 3.25 mm) depending on your individual crocheting tension

yarn needle

PATTERN STITCHES

ch, sl st, sc, Romanian lace cord stitch

LET ME SHOW YOU

Step 1: ch 2

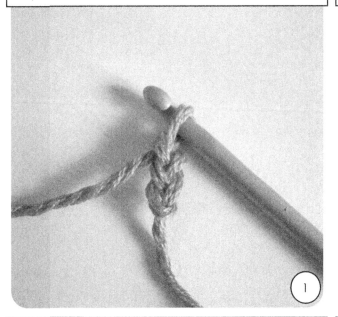

Step 2: sc 1 into the first ch (i.e. the 2nd ch from the hook)

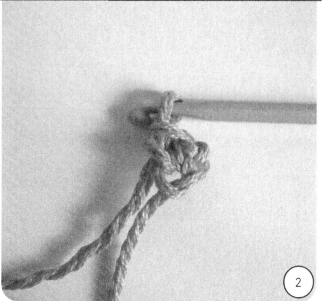

Step 3: flip your work clockwise (right to left) then *sc through the two loops formed by the previous stitch, positioned obliquely on the left side edge of your work*

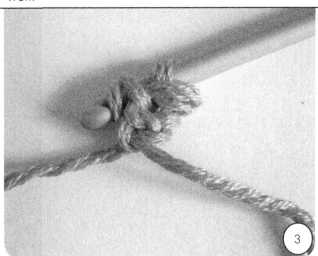

Step 4: keep flipping your work clockwise (right to left) and rep from *to*

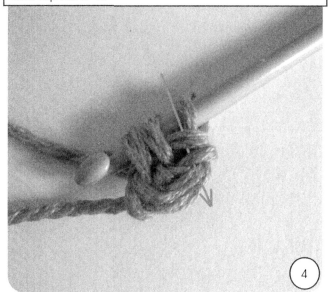

Step 5: Make a Romanian lace cord long enough to fit the pet (or the person) you are making it for.
Attach one little five-petal flower to one end of the Romanian lace cord.

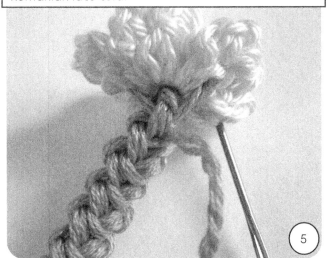

Step 6: Cut yarn and fasten off.

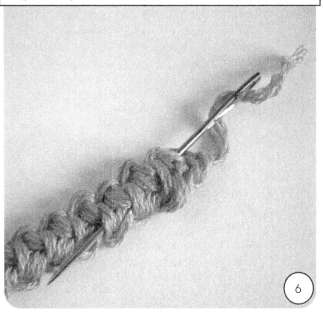

Step 7: With your yarn needle and the green cotton thread, fasten the flowers onto the cord. To do so, position the flower onto the cord and embroider 5 straight stitches going from the center of each flower into the middle of the petals, forming a star. As you form each straight stitch, catch in the Romanian lace cord underneath with your needle as well, pulling firmly on the thread to ensure the flower holds safely in place.

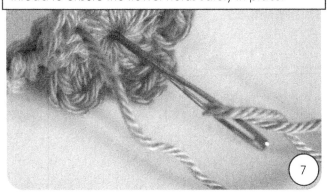

Step 8: You can embroider the flowers onto the cord alongside one another forming a row, or you can position them and embroider them on to your liking.

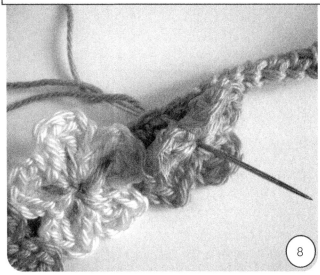

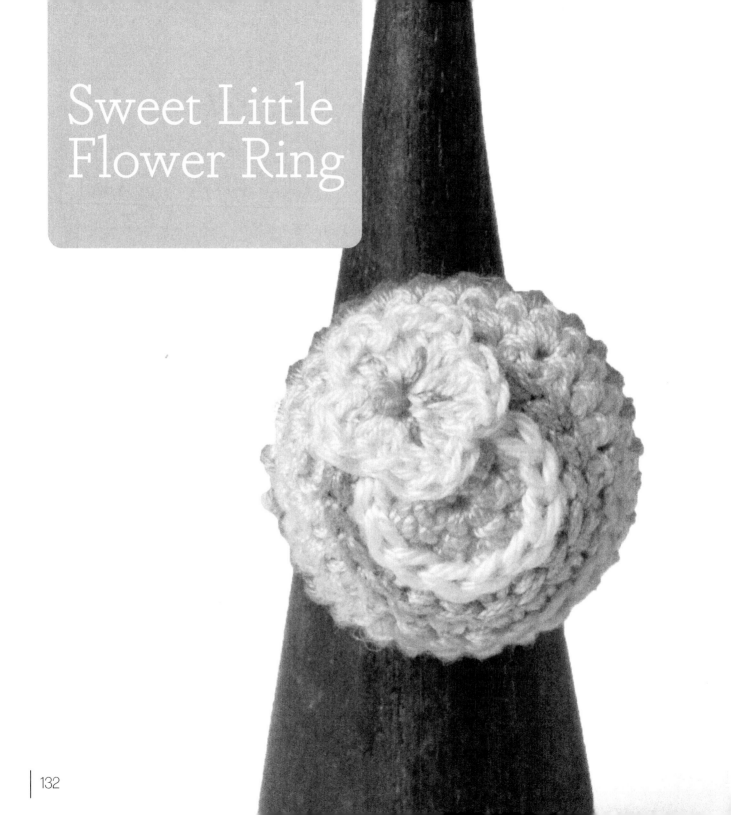

Sweet Little Flower Ring

Sweet Little Flower Ring

MATERIALS

SUPER FINE (1) weight (1.75 oz = 191 yards /50 g = 175 m) 100% high quality mercerized cotton thread: a total of about 1/3 of an oz (± 10 g) is required, made up of the following colors: turquoise, pink, light pink, dark green, light green, fuchsia, light blue.

steel hook size 4/0 (1.75 mm) or size 8 (1.50 mm), depending on your individual crocheting tension

yarn needle

fiber-fill or toy stuffing

1 five-petal flower in color to your liking

1 metal ring (select shape, style, color, wire thickness and material to your liking).

PATTERN STITCHES

crochet: ch, sl st, sc, dc2tog

embroidery: chain stitch, straight stitch, bullion knot stitch

PATTERN NOTES

The ring is composed of one embroidered crochet bead. The crochet bead is made up of 2 sections crocheted separately (front and rear). The front is embroidered and decorated, the sections (front and rear) are then join together in the course of the project.

The embroidered crochet bead is then attached to the metal ring.

INSTRUCTIONS

Step 1

FRONT (section 1)

With the pink, form a double loop and insert hook. Proceed as follows, ending each round with a sl st:

RND 1: ch 1, sc 6, pull firmly on the loop thread to close the starting loop.

RND 2: ch 1, sc 2 in each stitch around (= 12 stitches).

Cut and fasten off thread.

Continue with the turquoise: sl st 1 to attach thread, then

RND 3: ch 1, *sc 1, sc 2 into the next stitch around*; rep from *to* for another 5 times (= 18 stitches).

RND 4: ch 1, *sc 1 into each of the next 2 stitches round, sc 2 into the following stitch around*; rep from *to* another 5 times (= 24 stitches).

RND 5: ch 1, *sc 1 into each of the next 3 stitches round, 2 sc into the following stitch around*; rep from *to* another 5 times (= 30 stitches).

Cut and fasten off thread.

Step 2

With the light green thread embroider a round of chain stitches (using either a tapestry needle or a crochet hook) between rounds 2 and round 3.

Step 3

With the dark green embroider a round of chain stitches (using either a tapestry needle or a crochet hook)

between rounds 3 and round 4.

Step 4

With the fuchsia thread, embroider only a partial round i.e. make about 12 chain stitches (using either a tapestry needle or a crochet hook) between rounds 4 and round 5 as illustrated.

With your yarn needle and the green cotton thread, fasten the five-petal flower in place onto the bead. To do so, embroider 5 straight stitches going from the center of the flower into the middle of the petals, forming a star. As you form each straight stitch, catch in the bead surface underneath with your needle as well, pulling firmly on the thread to ensure the flower holds safely in place. Repeat with the light blue thread, alternating the light blue straight stitches to the green ones.

Complete your decoration with a bullion knot stitch.

Step 5

REAR (section 2)

With the turquoise, follow the same instructions given for the front of this bead, working round 1 to round 5 all in the same color.

Step 6

Crochet the two sections together (as instructed in Steps 1 to 4 on page 26).

Before closing the bead completely, roll a sufficient amount of fiber fill into a small, tight ball and fill the bead. Cut and fasten off thread.

ASSEMBLY

Sew the embroidered crochet bead onto the metal ring.

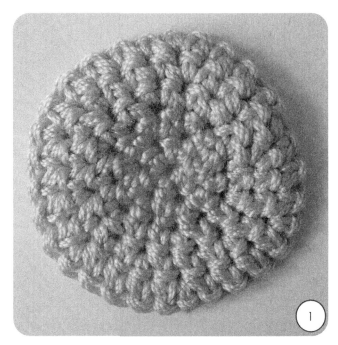

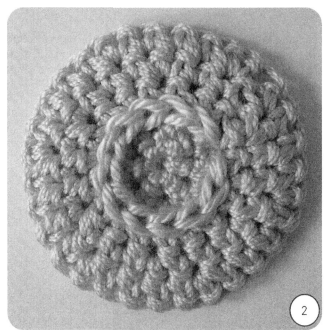

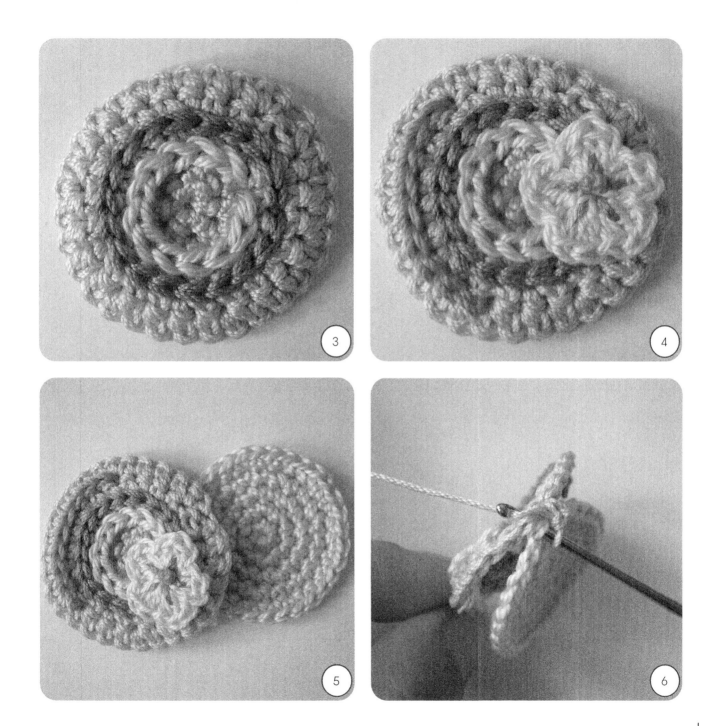

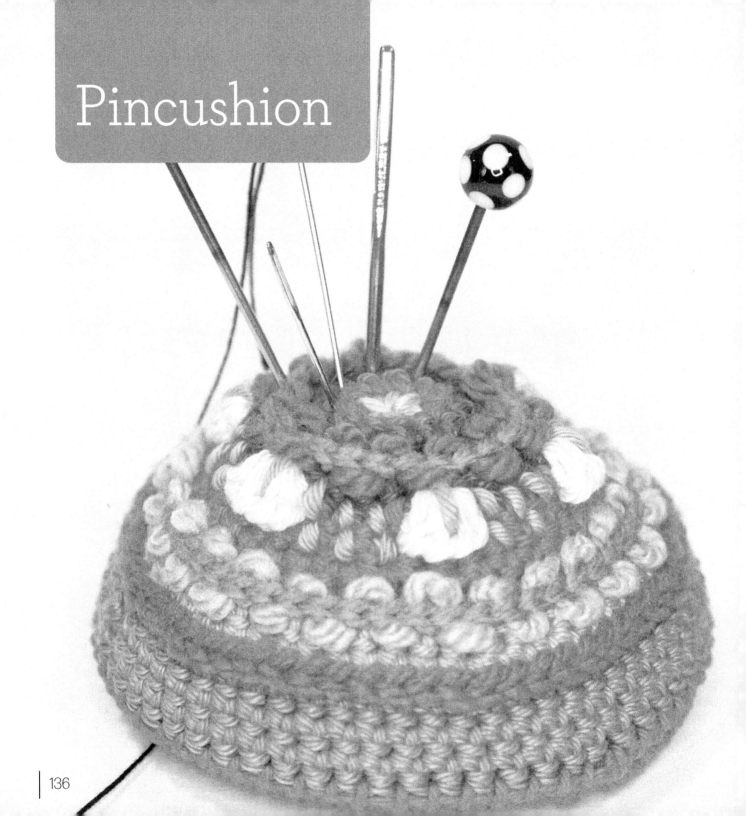

Pincushion

Pincushion

MATERIALS

Use your yarn leftovers and scraps!

100% cotton | fine (2) weight yarn (1.75oz = 137yds / 50g = 125m), about half an oz (15 g) in each of the following colors: red, purple, pink, green, bright yellow

Additional lengths (approx. 35") of 100% cotton crochet thread or embroidery floss in each of the following colors: turquoise, pink, light green, cyclamen purple

crochet hook sizes from a C-2 to a D-3 (2.75 to 3.25 mm) depending on your individual crocheting tension

yarn needle

fiber-fill or toy stuffing

a piece of thick red felt with a stiff finish

PATTERN STITCHES

crochet: ch, sl st, sc

embroidery: straight stitch, chain stitch, woven chain stitch, buttonhole stitch

PATTERN NOTES

The pincushion is made up of 2 sections, a crocheted top section and red felt underside section. The top section is embroidered, then both sections are joined together with an embroidered buttonhole stitch in the course of the project.

INSTRUCTIONS
TOP SECTION

Step 1

With the red yarn, form a double loop and insert hook. Proceed as follows, ending each round with a sl st:

RND 1: ch 1, sc 6, pull firmly on the loop yarn to close the starting loop.

RND 2: ch 1, 2 sc in each stitch around (= 12 stitches). Cut and fasten off yarn.

Step 2

Continue with the purple yarn: sl st 1 to attach yarn, then

RND 3: ch 1, *sc 1, sc 2 into the next stitch around*; rep from *to* for another 5 times (= 18 stitches).

RND 4: ch 1, *sc 1 into each of the next 2 stitches round, sc 2 into the following stitch around*; rep from *to* another 5 times (= 24 stitches).

LET ME SHOW YOU

RND 5: ch 1, *sc 1 into each of the next 3 stitches round, 2 sc into the following stitch around*; rep from *to* another 5 times (= 30 stitches).
Cut and fasten off yarn.

Step 3

Continue with the red:
RND 6: *1 sc completed with the bright yellow thread, make 1 bright yellow bobble stitch into the next stitch, completing this bo st with the red,
1 sc into each of the following 3 stitches*; rep *to* for another 5 times.
Cut and fasten off red yarn. Continue with the red.
RND 7: ch 1, *sc 1, sc 2 into the next stitch (1 increase), sc 1 into each of the following 3 stitches*, rep from *to* another 5 times (36 stitches).
RND 8: ch 1, *sc 1 into each of the following 5 stitches, sc 2 into the next stitch (1 increase)* rep from *to* another 5 times (42 stitches).
RND 9: ch 1, sc 1 into each of the following 2 stitches, *sc 2 into the next stitch (1 increase), sc 1 into each of the following 4 stitches*, rep from *to* another 5 times (48 stitches).
Cut and fasten off yarn.

Step 4

Continue with the pink:
RND 10: ch 1, *sc 1 into each of the following 7 stitches, sc 2 into the next stitch (1 increase)* rep *to* for another 5 times (54 stitches).
RND 11: ch 1, sc 1 into each of the following 3 stitches, *sc 2 into the next stitch (1 increase), sc 1 into each of the following 5 stitches*, rep from *to* another 5 times (48 stitches).

Cut and fasten off yarn.

Step 5

Continue with the green:
RND 12, 13, 14: ch 1, sc 1 into each stitch around (54 stitches).
Cut and fasten off yarn.

Step 6

With the light green thread, embroider seven straight stitches going from the center of the circle into the spaces between the top of each sc in the first round, to form a star.
With the pink thread, embroider straight stitches going from the 6th round into the 7th round.

Steps 7 & 8

With the turquoise thread (for chaining) and the cyclamen purple thread (for weaving), embroider a round of woven chain stitches between rounds 4 and round 5.
Do the chain stitches using either a tapestry needle or a crochet hook.
Use the cyclamen purple thread to do the weaving through the turquoise chain stitches.

With the turquoise (for chaining) and the light green thread (for weaving), embroider a round of woven chain stitches between rounds 9 and round 10.
Do the chain stitches using either a tapestry needle or a crochet hook.
Use cyclamen purple thread to do the weaving through the turquoise chain stitches.
With the cyclamen purple embroider a round of chain stitches between rounds 11 and round 12.

Step 9
Before embroidery and after embroidery

Step 10
UNDERSIDE SECTION
Place the bottom edge of the embroidered top section, front surface facing upwards, onto the red felt.
Carefully trace and then cut out a circle that neatly covers the underside.

Holding the bottom edge of the embroidered top section in position on the red felt circle underside, secure the edges of the two sections together with a basic buttonhole stitch as follows:
with a yarn needle and a length of yarn that is heavier than the yarn used for the crochet top section, bring needle out at starting point along edge. *Measure one stitch-gap away,
put needle in from front to back in the gap between the last two crochet rounds perpendicular to this point (through both the top and the underside sections), bring needle out and hold it in position (one stitch-gap away) under the edge at right angles from entry point without pulling it out completely. Pull the working yarn under the protruding needle point and then wind it completely around the needle once in a circular, clockwise motion. Pull the needle out completely so that the yarn tightens forming a perpendicular straight stitch with a small knot in the yarn running along the edge*.
Repeat * to * in all stitch gaps around top section, minding that you leave a large enough opening for filling before completing all stitches. Cut and fasten off yarn.

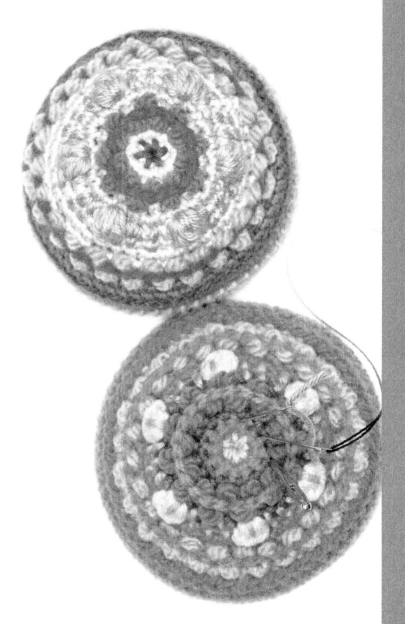

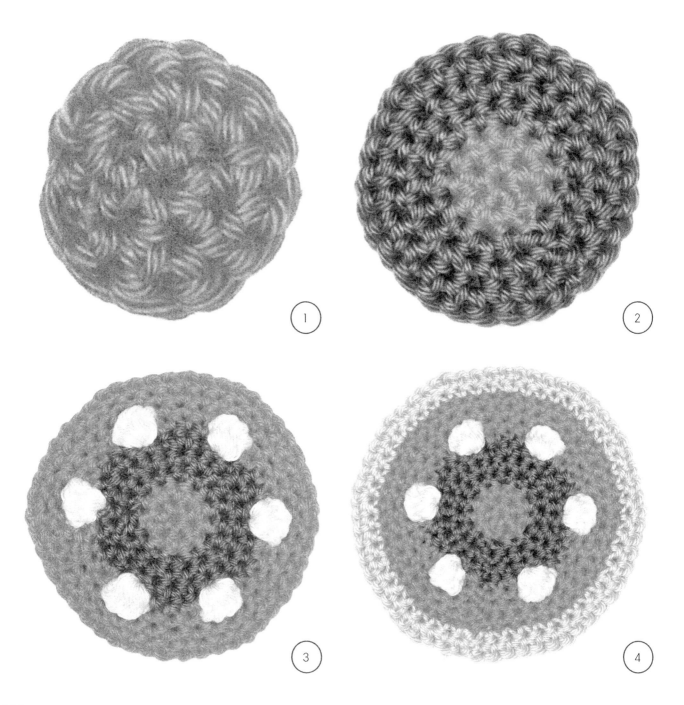

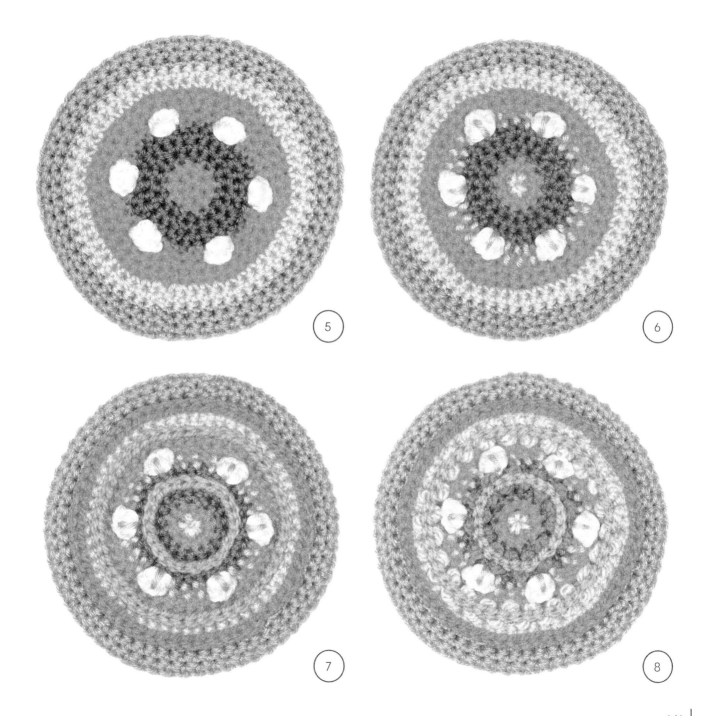

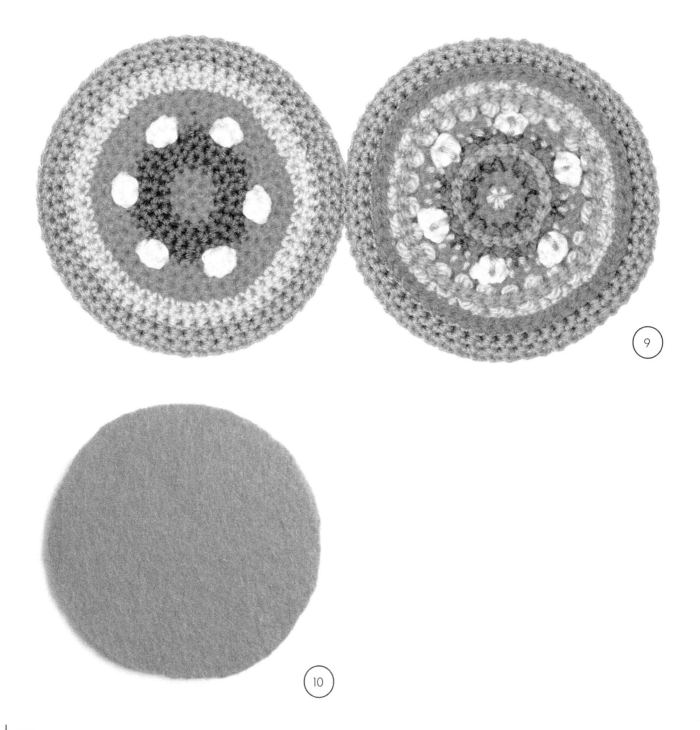

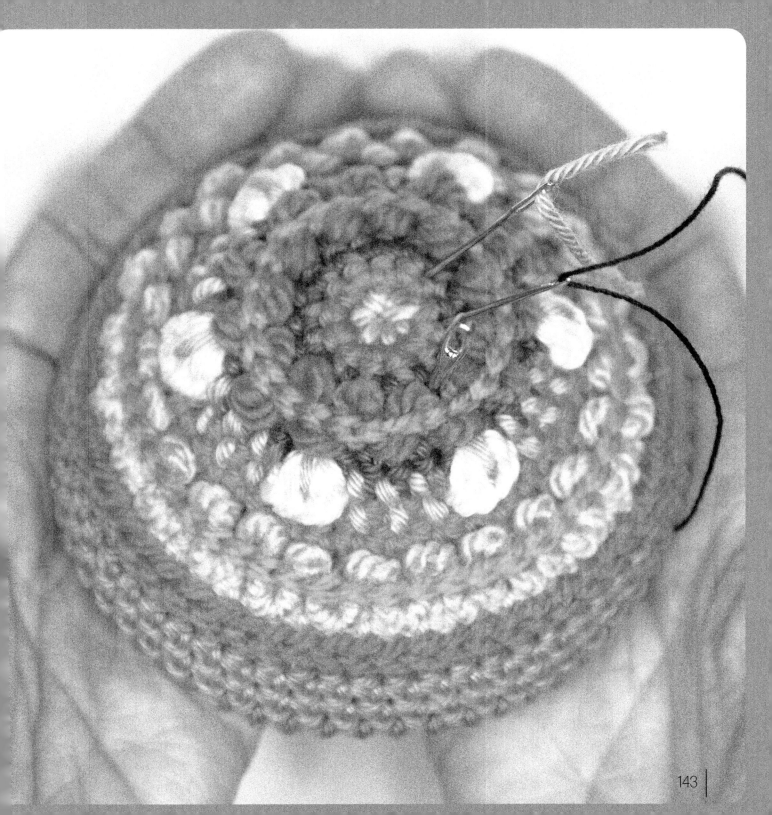

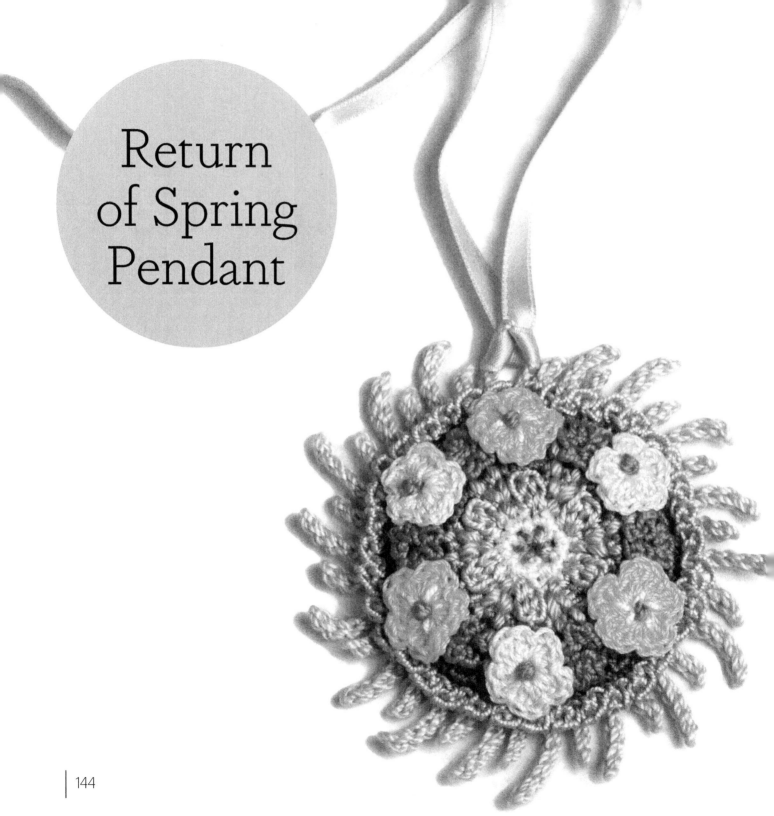

Return
of Spring
Pendant

Return of Spring Pendant

MATERIALS

SUPER FINE (1) weight (1.75 oz = 191 yards /50 g = 175 m) 100% high quality mercerized cotton thread:

a total of about 1/3 of an oz (± 10 g) is required, made up of the following colors:

brown, mustard yellow, bright yellow, turquoise, cyclamen purple.

A total of 6 five-petal flowers (made as instructed in Steps 1 to 6 on page...) 3 in fuchsia and 3 in light pink

A few additional threads, each approx. 30" (75 cm) long, color wisteria violet

steel hook size 4/0 (1.75 mm) or size 8 (1.50 mm), depending on your individual crocheting tension

yarn needle

fiber-fill or toy stuffing (or a large, flat shaped button)

PATTERN STITCHES

crochet: ch, sl st, sc, sc in front loop, sc in back loop

decorative fringe stitch: ch 4(5,6,7,8) insert hook into 2nd chain from hook and 1 sl st into each one of the following ch)

embroidery: chain stitch (or surface crochet slip stitch), straight stitch, bullion knot stitch

PATTERN NOTES

The pendant is composed of one embroidered crochet bead. The crochet bead is made up of 2 sections crocheted separately (front and rear).

The front is embroidered and decorated, the sections (front and rear) are then joined together in the course of the project.

LET ME SHOW YOU

INSTRUCTIONS

Step 1
FRONT (SECTION 1)

With the bright yellow, form a double loop and insert hook. Proceed as follows, ending each round with a sl st:
RND 1: ch 1, sc 6, pull firmly on the loop thread to close the starting loop.
RND 2: ch 1, sc 2 in each stitch around (= 12 stitches).
Cut and fasten off thread.

Step 2

Continue with the mustard yellow: sl st 1 to attach thread, then
RND 3: ch 1, *sc 1, sc 2 into the next stitch around*; rep from *to* for another 5 times (= 18 stitches).
RND 4: ch 1, *sc 1 into each of the next 2 stitches round, sc 2 into the following stitch around*; rep from *to* another 5 times (= 24 stitches).
Cut and fasten off thread.

Step 3

Continue with the brown: sl st 1 to attach thread, then
RND 5: ch 1, *sc 1 into each of the next 3 stitches round, 2 sc into the following stitch around*; rep from *to* another 5 times (= 30 stitches).
RND 6: *sc 1, sc 2 into the next stitch (1 increase), sc 1 into each of the following 3 stitches*, rep from *to* another 5 times (36 stitches).
RND 7 and 8: sc 1 into each stitch around, sl st 1 to close round.
Cut yarn and fasten off.

Step 4

Continue with the turquoise: sl st 1 to attach thread, then
RND 9: *sc in front loop 1 and ch 3 in next stitch*; rep from *to* to the end of the round. Cut and fasten off yarn.

Step 5

With the cyclamen purple thread embroider 6 straight stitches going from the center of the circle into the spaces between the top of each sc in the first round, to form a star.
With the turquoise thread, embroider a petal of chain stitches between round 3 and round 4 for a total of 6 petals.
With the wisteria violet thread, embroider straight stitches going from the 3rd round into the 4th round and going from the 4rd round into the 5th round,
to form a series of small "Ys" through the the sc increases made in the round 4.
With the cyclamen purple thread, embroider a round of chain stitches (using either a needle or a crochet hook) between round 5 and round 8.

With your yarn needle and the bright yellow cotton thread, fasten the five-petal flower in place onto the bead. To do so, embroider 5 straight stitches going from the center of the flower into the middle of the petals, forming a star.
As you form each straight stitch, catch in the bead surface underneath with your needle as well, pulling firmly on the thread to ensure the flower holds safely in place.
Complete your decoration with a bullion knot stitch.

REAR (SECTION 2)

With the brown, follow the same instructions given for the front of this bead, working round 1 to round 8 all in the same color. Cut and fasten off yarn.

ASSEMBLY

Place back of section 2 against back of section 1 and crochet the two sections together as follows:

With the pink sl st 1 to attach thread, then *insert hook into both the next stitch of section 2 and directly into the corresponding back loop stitch of section 1, to sc 1, decorative fringe 1*. Repeat to join all stitches round.

Before closing the bead completely, fill the bead. Cut and fasten off thread.

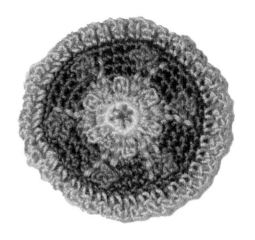

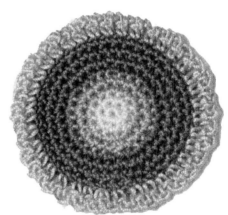

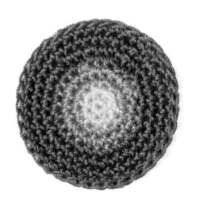

Return of Spring Pendant

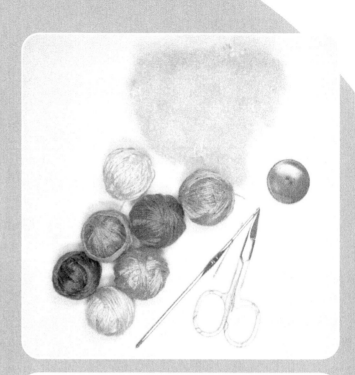

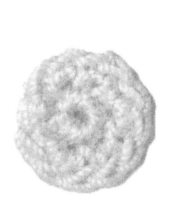

①

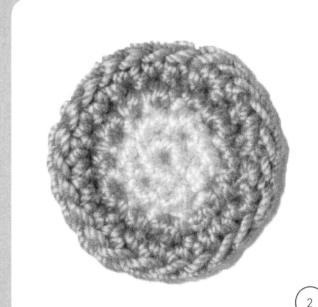

②

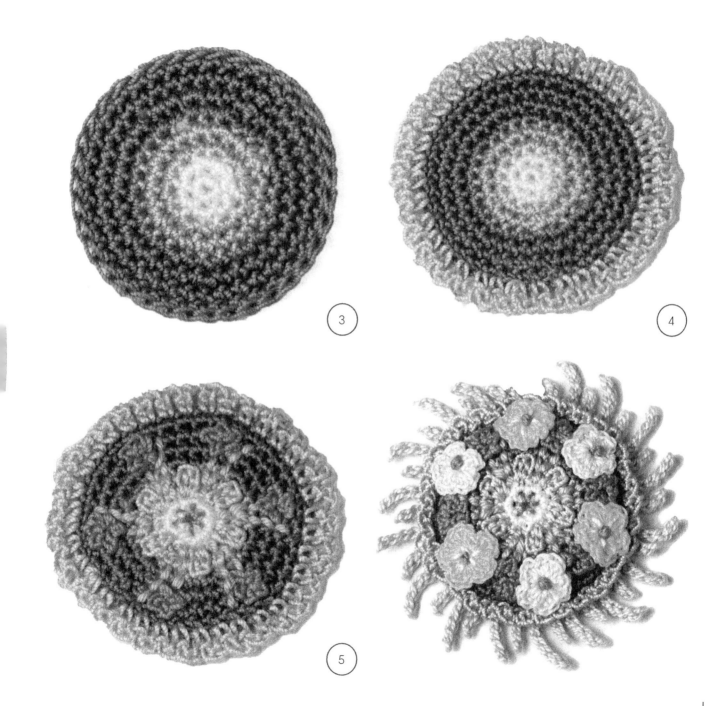

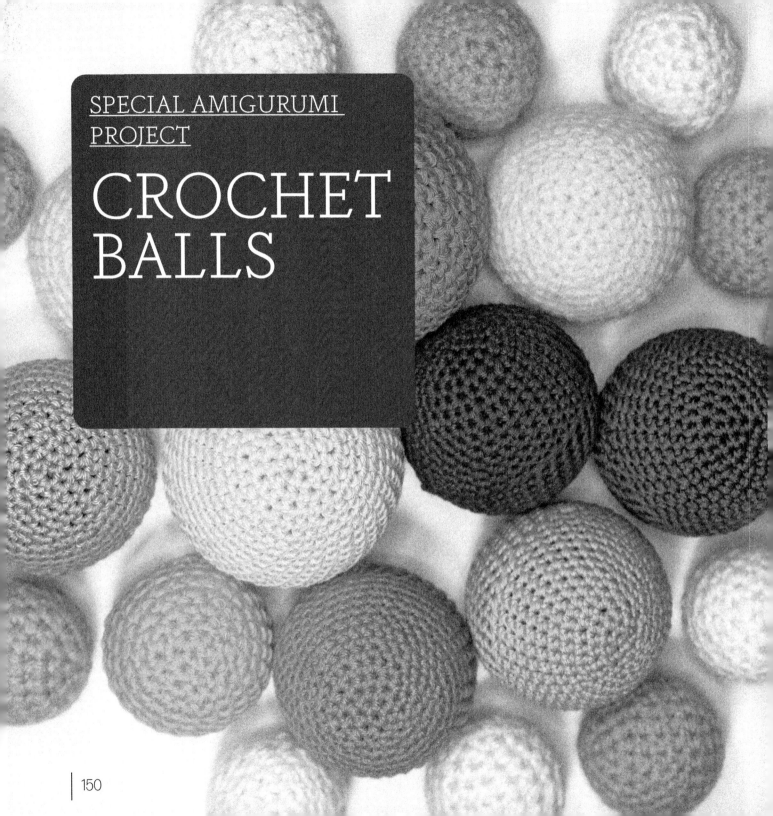

CROCHET BALLS

Your First
AMIGURUMI

Are you ready to start your journey into the magical world of 3D amigurumi crochet projects?
Your amigurumi journey starts from a simple and playful crochet ball.

LET'S GET STARTED!!

LET ME SHOW YOU

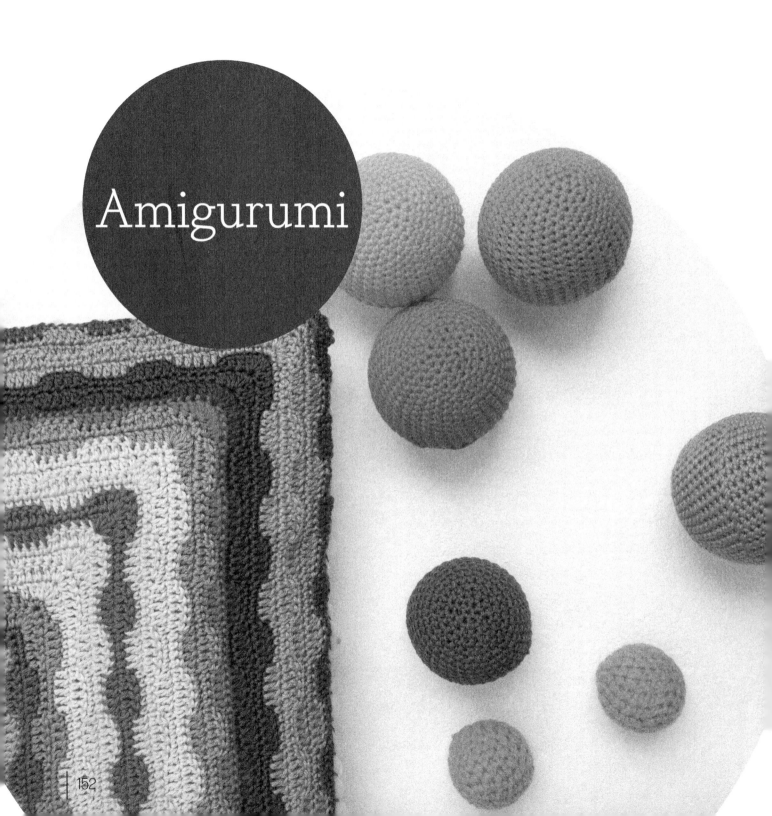

Amigurumi

Crochet Balls

MATERIALS

about 1oz (30 g) 100% cotton | fine (2) weight yarn (1.75oz = 137yds / 50g = 125m) color: bright blue
crochet hook C-2 or D-3 (3.25 – 3.75 mm)
yarn needle
1 plastic ball having a diameter of 4" (10 cm) or synthetic fiber-fill

PATTERN STITCHES

ch, sl st, sc

INSTRUCTIONS

STEP 1

section 1: follow the instructions given for the polka dots (RND 1 - 8)

STEP 2

RND 9, 10, 11 and 12: sc 1 into each stitch around, sl st 1 to close round. Cut yarn and fasten off.

STEP 3

section 2: follow the same instruction given for the section 1 and cut and fasten off the yarn leaving an end approx. 10 inches (25 cm) long. Sew the two sections (insert the yarn needle in 1 sc into each stitch around section 1 the corresponding stitch around the the section 2)

STEP 4

While sewing the two sections insert the plastic ball (or stuff with the fiber-fill).

A tip for crocheters wishing to begin making 3D crochet sculptures for the first time.
I suggest starting out with a sphere: in amigurumi crochet it's important to learn how to make decreases and increases. Balls require a lot of exercising this skills. The next step will be a crochet heart. Then a further step will be making different pieces and putting them together.
I will lead you through this journey, so come along with me!

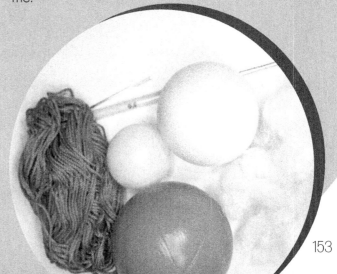

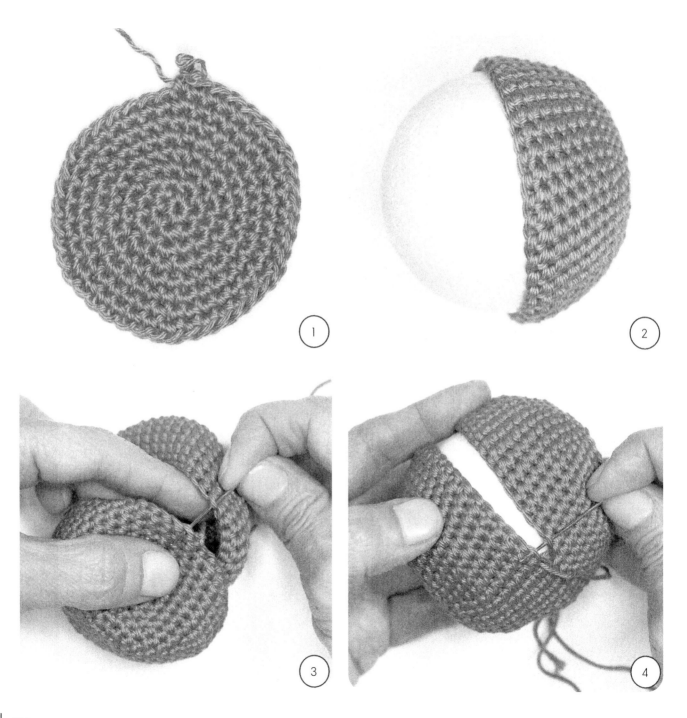

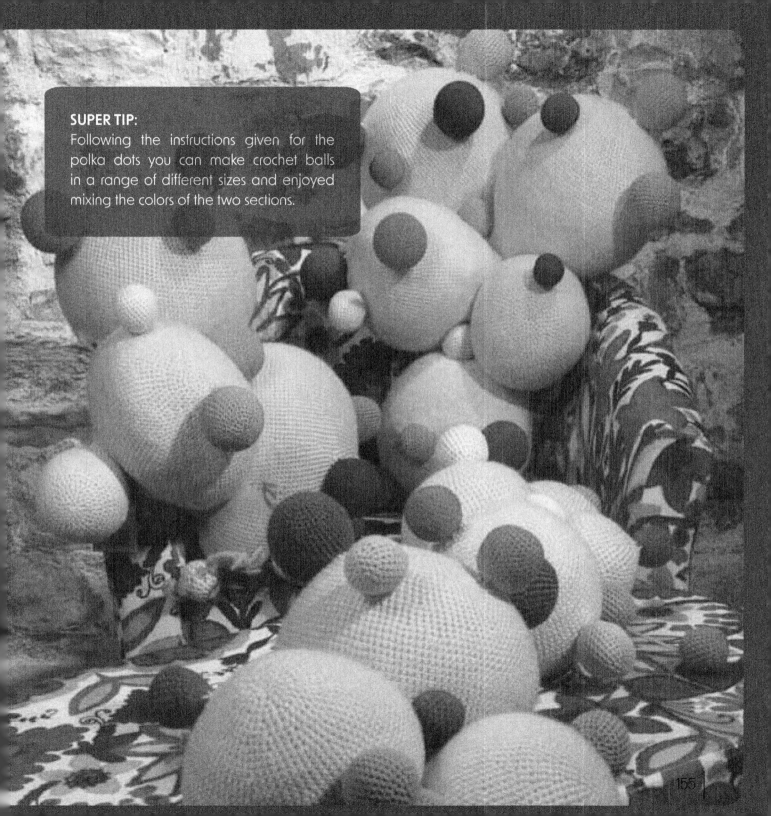

SUPER TIP:
Following the instructions given for the polka dots you can make crochet balls in a range of different sizes and enjoyed mixing the colors of the two sections.

3D CROCHET HEART

3D Crochet Heart

This heart is made up starting with two upper cup sections that are crocheted separately and then joined together to form the bottom tip section

MATERIALS

100% cotton | fine (2) weight yarn (1.75oz = 137yds / 50g = 125m)
1,75 oz (50 g)
crochet hook C-2 or D-3 (3.25 – 3.75 mm)
yarn needle
fiber- fill or toy stuffing

PATTERN STITCHES

ch, sl st, sc

SUPER TIP: you can make different sized 3D hearts simply by changing the size of the upper cup sections.
Always ensure that both cup sections are identical to one another: to do so count the number of stitches in the last round of each section (the stitch count should be identical) before joining them together.

INSTRUCTIONS

STEP 1

For the first cup section, form a double loop and insert hook
RND 1: ch 1, sc 6.
RND 2: *sc 2 in each stitch*, rep from *to* another 5 times (12 stitches).
RND 3: *sc 1, sc 2 in the following stitch (1 increase)*; rep from *to* another 5 times (18 stitches).
RND 4: *sc 2 in next stitch (1 increase), sc 1 in following 2 stitches*; rep from *to* another 5 times (24 stitches).
RND 5: *sc 1 into each of the following 3 stitches, sc 2 into the next stitch (1 increase)* rep from *to* another 5 times (30 stitches).

STEP 2

RND 6, 7, 8, 9: sc 1 into each stitch around. Sl st 1 to close round, cut yarn and fasten off.

STEP 3

For the second cup section, follow the same instructions given for the first but do not cut yarn after round 9, so that you have one loop left on your hook.

LET ME SHOW YOU

STEP 4

To join the two cup sections together, place them one alongside the other as illustrated. With the inside of cup section 2 facing you and your one loop already on hook, insert hook simultaneously through the next stitch in cup section 2 and a corresponding sc stitch in cup section 1, then sc 1.

STEP 5

Make another 5 sc in the same manner over the next 5 stitches. This forms a neat central seam that firmly holds the two cup sections together.

STEP 6

With the inside of cup section 2 facing you continue making sc 1 into each of the next 23 stitches

STEP 7

insert hook into the last stitch of cup section 2, yarn over and draw up a loop

STEP 8

insert hook into the first stitch of cup section 1, yarn over and draw up a loop

STEP 9

you now have 3 loops on your hook, yarn over and draw through all 3 loops on hook (1 decrease)

STEP 10

sc 1 into the next 22 stitches around, decrease 1.

STEP 11

sc 1 into the next 21 stitches around,

STEP 12

insert hook into the following stitch, yarn over and draw up a loop, insert hook into the following stitch, yarn over and draw up a loop, insert hook into the following stitch, yarn over and draw up a loop: you now have 4 loops on your hook

STEP 13

yarn over and draw through all 4 loops on hook (2 decreases)

STEP 14

sc 1 into the next 20 stitches around, decrease 2, sc 1 into the next 18 stitches, decrease 2.

TIP: as you crochet on and the opening grows smaller, gradually keep stuffing the heart with fiber-fill.

Proceed crocheting in spiral rounds as follows, always working in 2 decreases on top of the decreases made in the previous round:

sc 1 in next 18, dec 2, sc 1 in next 17, dec 2,
sc 1 in next 16, dec 2, sc 1 in next 15, dec 2,
sc 1 in next 14, dec 2, sc 1 in next 13, dec 2,
sc 1 in next 12, dec 2, sc 1 in next 11, dec 2,
sc 1 in next 10, dec 2, sc 1 in next 9, dec 2,
sc 1 in next 8, dec 2, sc 1 in next 7, dec 2,
sc 1 in next 6, dec 2, sc 1 in next 5, dec 2,
sc 1 in next 4, dec 2, sc 1 in next 3, dec 2,
sc 1 in next 2, dec 2, sc 1, dec 2,
dec 2, cut and fasten off yarn.

Amigurumi

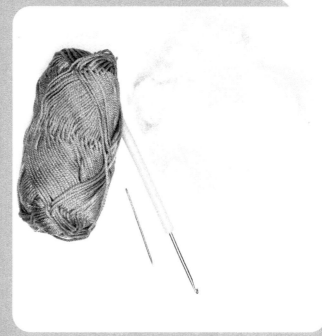

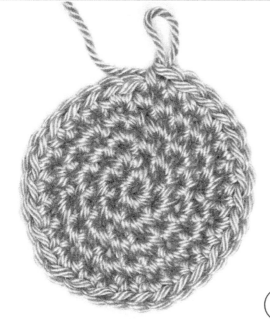

①

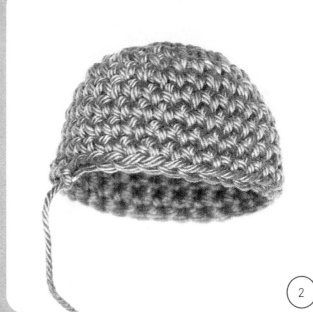

②

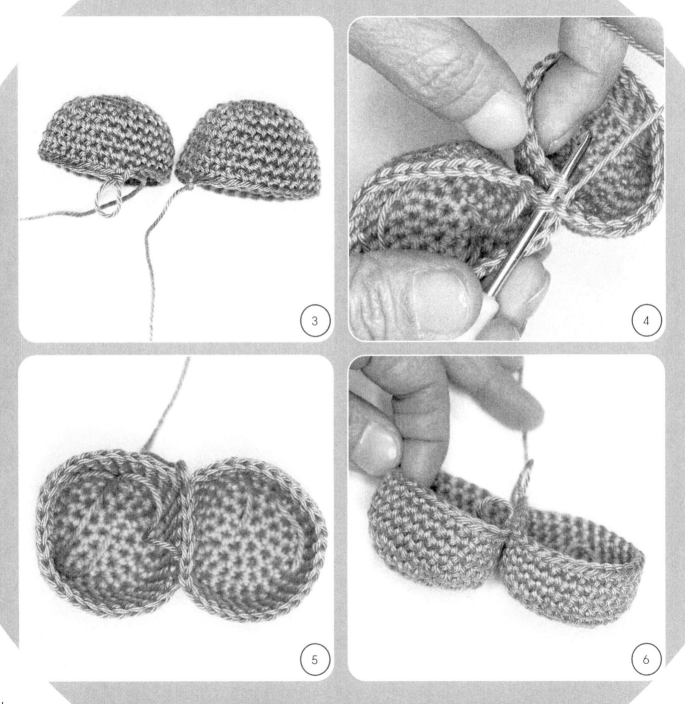

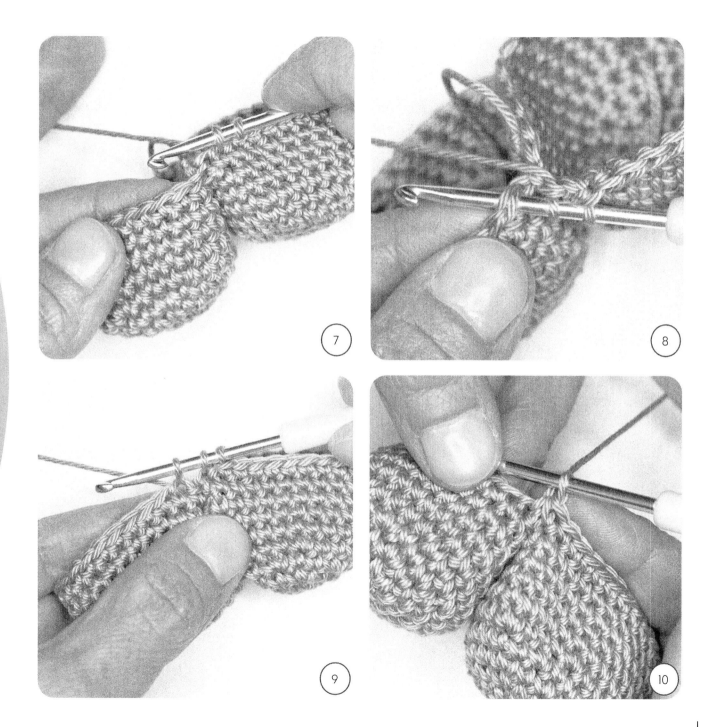

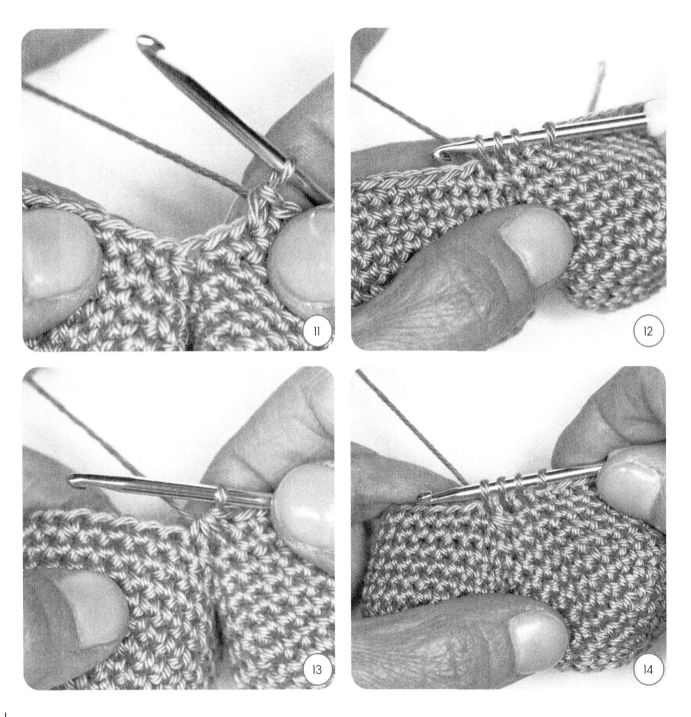

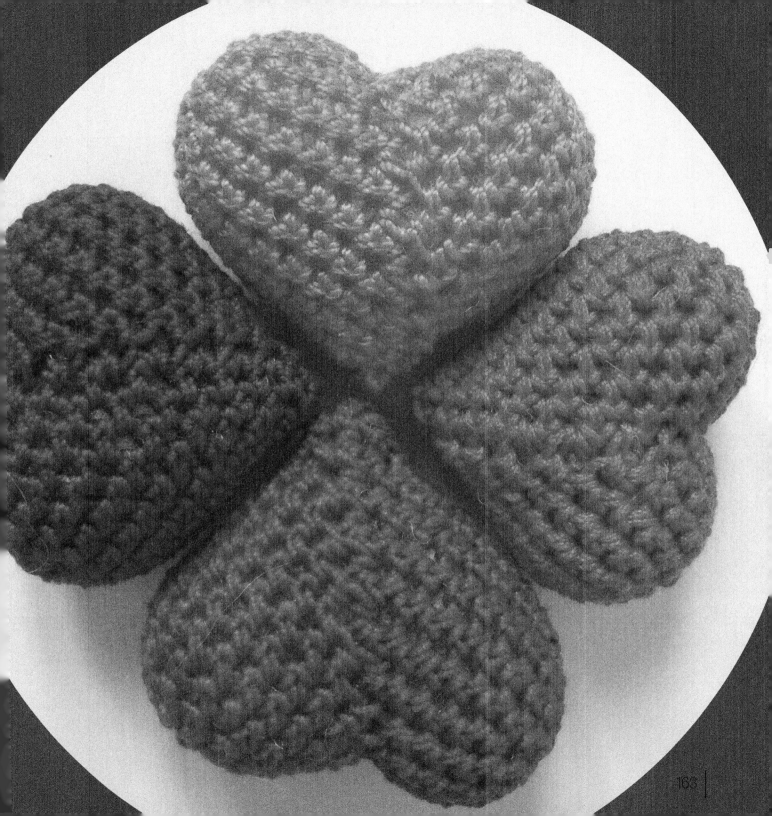

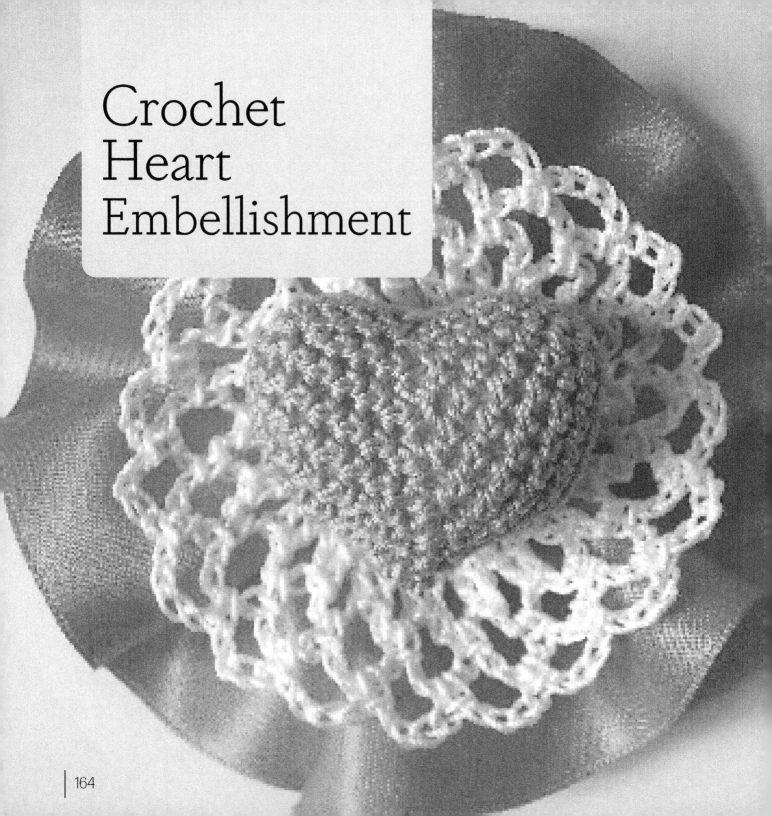

Crochet Heart Embellishment

Crochet Heart Embellishment

MATERIALS

1 small crochet heart
satin ribbon 20" (50 cm) long, 4" (10 cm) high
1 recycled lace doily having a diameter of 3" (8 cm)
sewing needle and sewing thread

STEP 2

Work a row of running stitches along one of the top edges of the ribbon.

STEP 3

Form into a rosette

STEP 4

Overlap the three elements as illustrated and sew them on reverse with tight, neat stitches so that they hold firmly together.

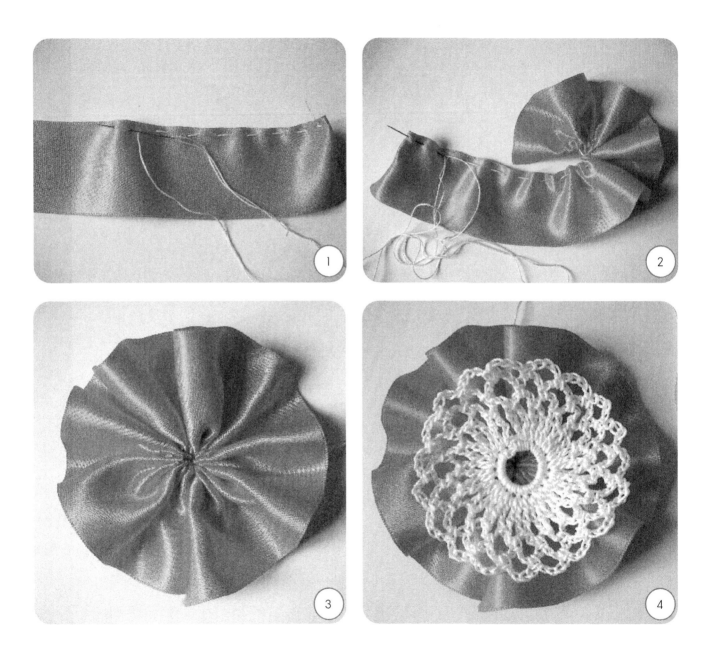

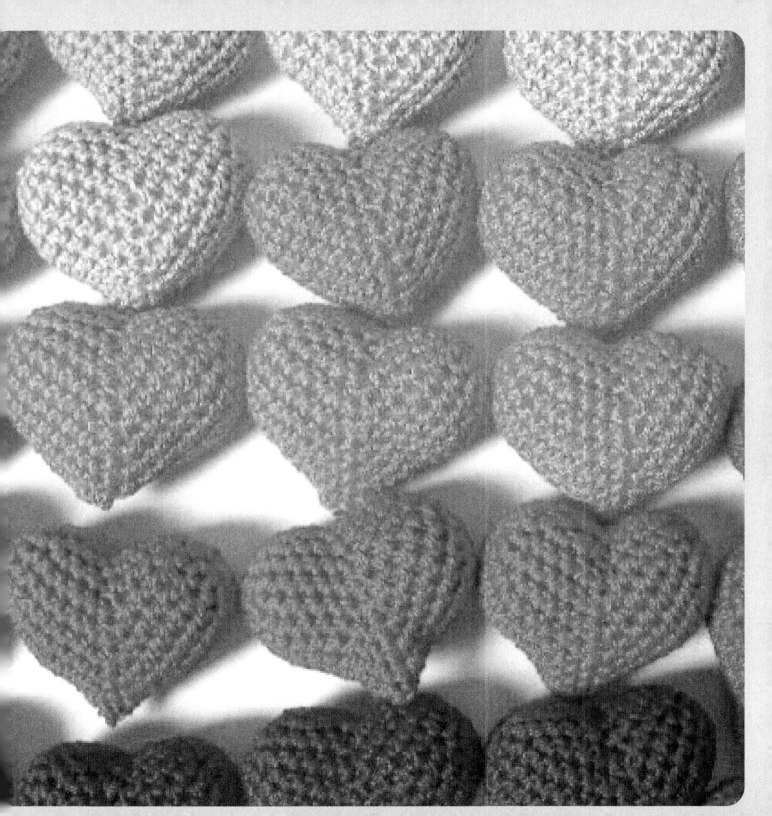

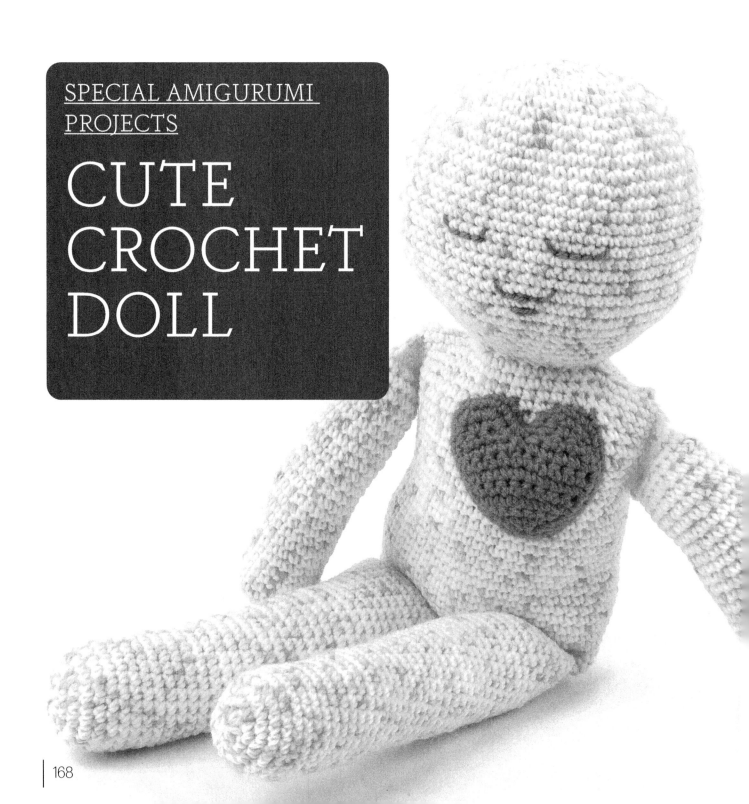

CUTE CROCHET DOLL

Cute Crochet Doll

SUPER TIP:

if you aren't advanced crocheters and you're wondering how to choose the right yarn for your doll, I recommend you start out using a heavier weight yarn. Your doll will work up quicker, even if you manage to crochet only a few rows a day. Obviously, using a thicker yarn will result in a bigger doll whereas a thinner yarn will result in a smaller sized doll.

I have made some really tiny dolls using exactly the same pattern with the same number of stitches and rows but using extra fine cotton lace weight thread, the same used for bobbin, tatting and crochet laces.

Therefore the appearance of your finished doll will change based on the different types of yarn weights you intend using.

MATERIALS

3.5 oz (100 g) light (3) weight yarn in a skin-toned color.
crochet hook size E-4 (3.50 mm)
yarn needle
fiber- fill or toy stuffing

LET ME SHOW YOU

PATTERN STITCHES

ch, sl st, sc

single crochet 2 together (decrease): insert hook into a stitch, yarn over and draw up a loop, insert hook into the following stitch, yarn over and draw up a loop - you now have 3 loops on your hook - yarn over and draw through all 3 loops on hook

single crochet in front loop only: make a single crochet inserting hook only into the front loop i.e. the loop that is closest to you of the 2 loops that make up the top V shape of a stitch.

INSTRUCTIONS

Step 1

For the first leg of the doll, form a double loop and insert hook, then work in tubular rounds as follows:

RND 1: ch 1, sc 8.

RND 2: *sc 1, sc 2 in the following stitch (1 increase)*; rep from *to* another 7 times (12 stitches).

RND 3: sc 2 in each stitch around (24 stitches).

RND 4 to RND 42: sc 1 into each stitch around. Sl st 1 to close round, cut yarn and fasten off.

Step 2

For the second leg of the doll, follow the same instructions given for the first but do not cut yarn after round 42, so that you have one loop left on your hook.

Step 3

Stuff both legs with fiber-fill or toy stuffing, then holding the top edges of the second leg together as shown, ch 2 (replaces first stitch),

insert hook through two corresponding top edge stitches (the first stitch and the matching stitch on back) and sc 1, repeat from * to * until top edge is closed.

Step 4

Don't cut yarn of second leg just closed but ch 2,

Step 5

repeat from * to * on first leg too until top edge is closed, turn your work.

Step 6

Ch 2 (replaces first stitch), sc 1 in each stitch across to end of row.

Step 7

In next row, ch 2, single crochet in front loop only (make a single crochet inserting hook only into the front loop i.e. the loop that is closest to you of the 2 loops that make up the top V shape of a stitch) in each stitch across.

Step 8

On completion of row, flip your work clockwise and sc 1 in each remaining loop of the same row.

Proceed with building up the body tube by working in tubular, single crochet rounds until you have 20 rounds.
RND 21: single crochet 2 together (decrease) six times to make 6 decreases, spacing them at regular intervals throughout this round.
RND 22 to RND32: sc 1 into each stitch around. Sl st 1 to close round, cut yarn and fasten off.

Step 9

For the arms of the doll, form a double loop and insert hook, then work in tubular rounds as follows:
RND 1: ch 1, sc 8.
RND 2: *sc 2 in each stitch*, rep from *to* another 7 times (16 stitches).
RND 3: *sc 3, sc 2 in the following stitch (1 increase)*; rep from *to* another 7 times (20 stitches).
RND 4 to RND 29: sc 1 into each stitch around. Sl st 1 to close round.

Step 10

Stuff the arm with fiber-fill or toy stuffing, then holding the top edges together as shown, ch 2 (replaces first stitch), *insert hook through two corresponding top edge stitches (the first stitch and the matching stitch on back) and sc 1*, repeat from * to * until top edge is closed.
Make 2.

Step 11

For the head of the doll form a double loop and insert hook, then work in tubular rounds as follows:
RND 1: ch 1, sc 8.
RND 2: *sc 2 in each stitch*, rep from *to* another 7 times (16 stitches).

RND 3: *sc 1, sc 2 in the following stitch (1 increase)*; rep from *to* another 7 times (24 stitches).

RND 4: *sc 2 in next stitch (1 increase), sc 1 in following 2 stitches*; rep from *to* another 7 times (32 stitches).

RND 5: sc 1 into each stitch around

RND 6: *sc 1 into each of the following 3 stitches, sc 2 into the next stitch (1 increase)* rep from *to* another 7 times (40 stitches).

RND 7: sc 1 into each stitch around

RND 8: sc 1, *sc 2 into the next stitch (1 increase), sc 1 into each of the following 4 stitches*, rep from *to* another 7 times (48 stitches).

RND 9: *sc 1 in following 2 stitches, sc 2 in next stitch (1 increase), *; rep from *to* another 7 times (64 stitches).

RND 10, 11: sc 1 into each stitch around

RND 12: *sc 1 into each of the following 7 stitches, sc 2 into the next stitch (1 increase)* rep *to* for another 7 times (72 stitches).

RND 13 to RND 25: sc 1 into each stitch around

RND 26: *sc 1 into each of the following 2 stitches, 1 decrease, *; rep from *to* another 7 times.

RND 27, 28, 29: sc 1 into each stitch around

RND 30: *sc 1 in following 2 stitches, 1 decrease, *; rep from *to* another 7 times.

RND 31: single crochet 2 together (decrease) five times to make 5 decreases, spacing them at regular intervals throughout this round.

Sl st 1 to close round. Stuff the head.

Step 12

You've completed the body sections of the doll.

Step 13

Stuff the body tube with fiber-fill or toy stuffing, then close it with a seam, leaving a 24-stitch opening for attaching the doll's head.

Please note: the opening needs to be of the appropriate width so that the head, once attached, holds up straight and doesn't fall. Since the head is self-sustained, a neck section is not required.

Step 14

Stuff the head with fiber-fill or toy stuffing and sew the head onto the 24-stitch opening in the body tube.

Step 15

Sew the arms to the body

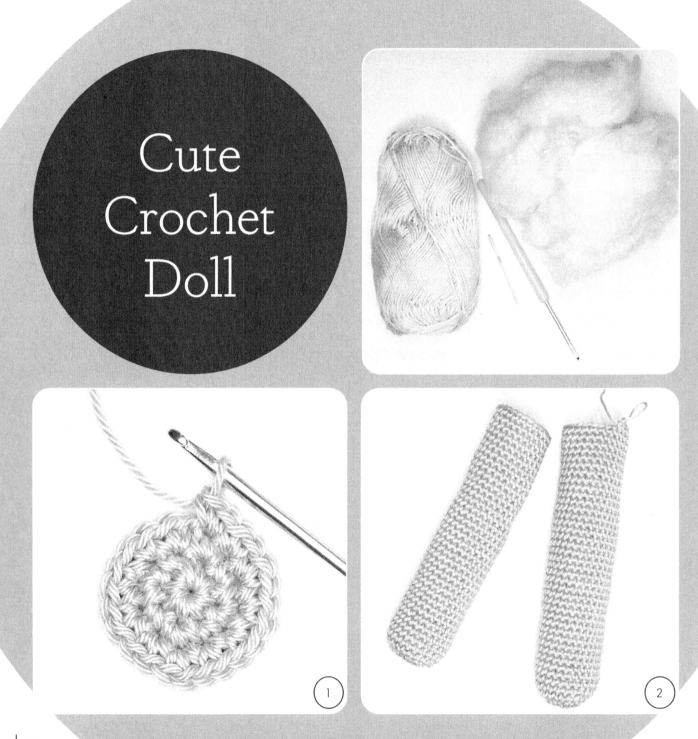

Cute Crochet Doll

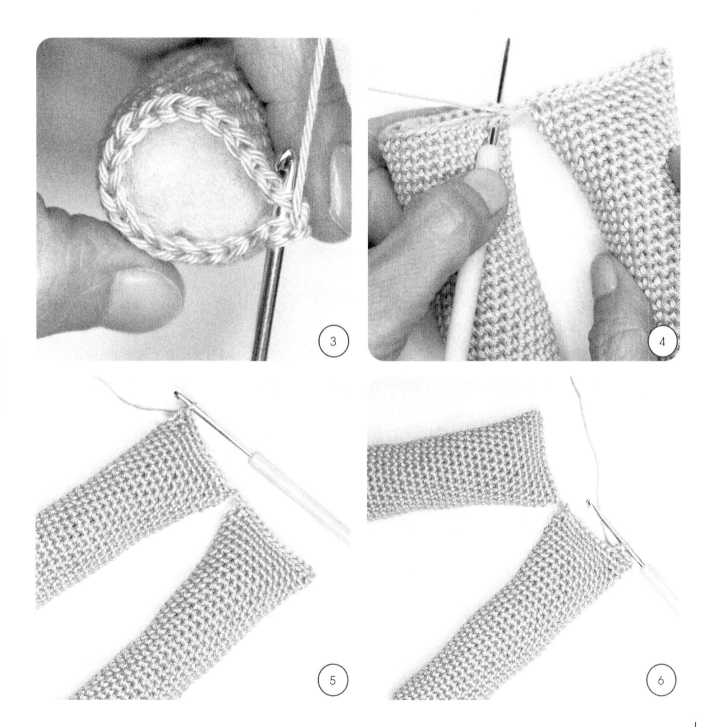

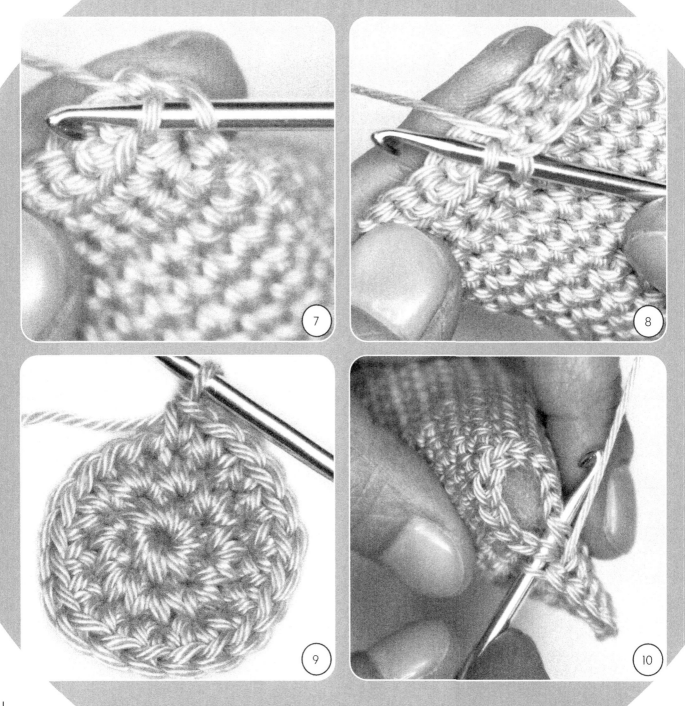

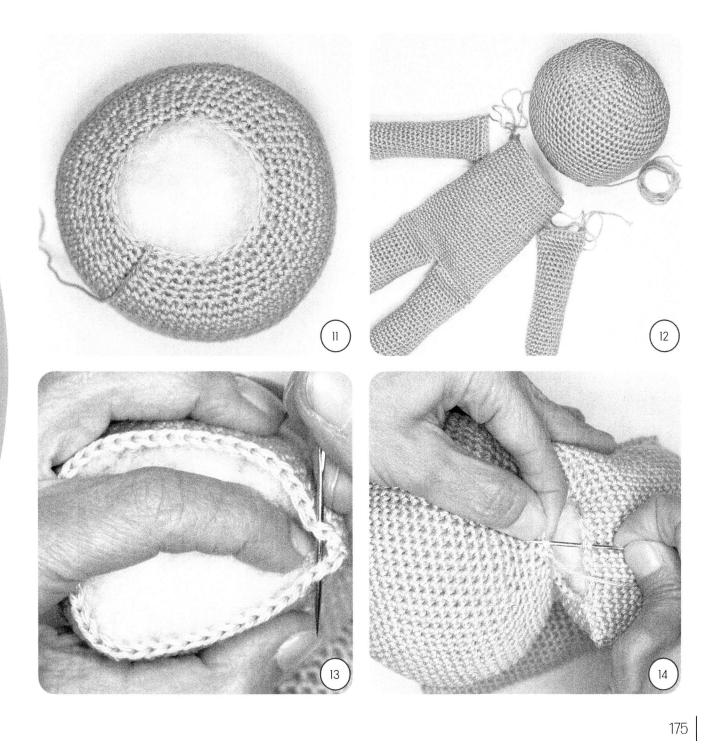

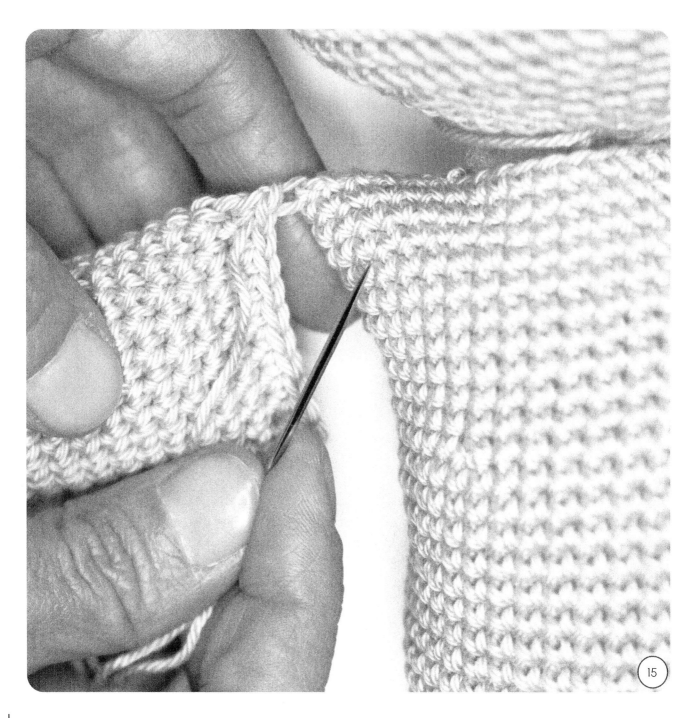

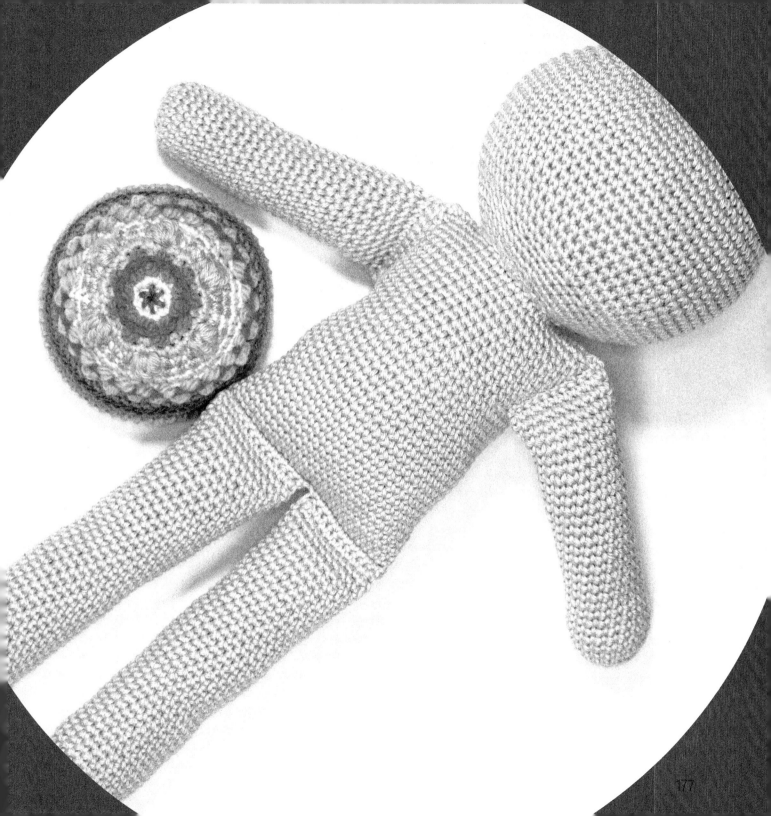

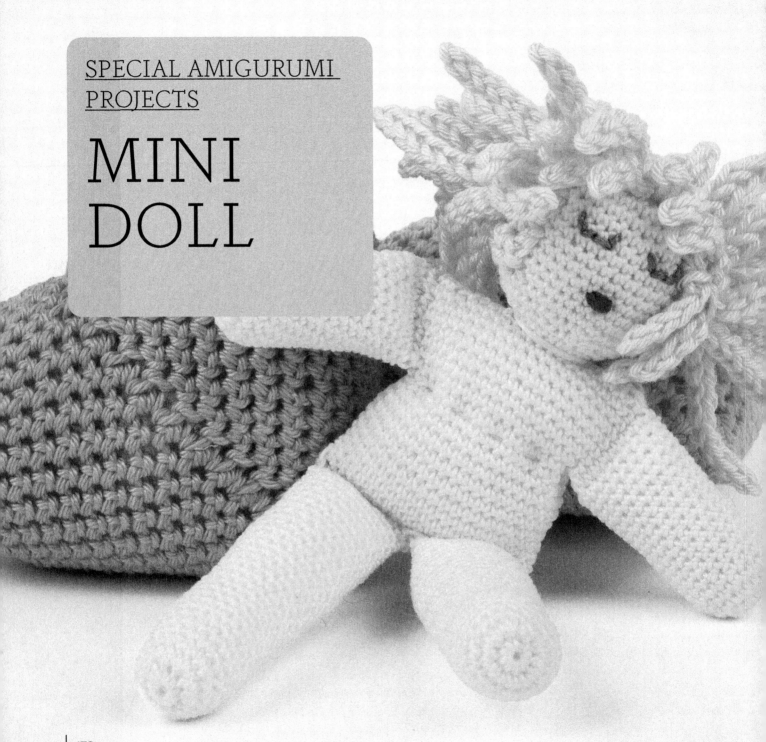

MINI DOLL

Mini Doll

MATERIALS

SUPER FINE (1) weight (1.75 oz = 213 yards /50 g = 195 m)
100% high quality mercerized cotton thread:
a total of about 0,80 oz (± 25 g) color: white
steel hook size 9/4 (1.25 mm) or size 7 (1.50 mm),
depending on your individual crocheting tension

SUPER FINE (1) weight (1.75 oz = 191 yards /50 g = 175 m)
100% high quality mercerized cotton thread:
about half an oz (± 15 g) is required in bright yellow
steel hook size 4/0 (1.75 mm) or size 8 (1.50 mm),
depending on your individual crocheting tension
yarn needle
fiber-fill or toy stuffing

PATTERN STITCHES

ch, sl st, sc

single crochet 2 together (decrease): insert hook into a
stitch, yarn over and draw up a loop, insert hook into
the following stitch, yarn over and draw up a loop - you
now have 3 loops on your hook - yarn over and draw
through all 3 loops on hook

single crochet in front loop only: make a single crochet
inserting hook only into the front loop i.e. the loop that
is closest to you of the 2 loops that make up the top V
shape of a stitch.

decorative fringe stitch: ch 4(5,6,7) insert hook into 2nd
chain from hook, sl st 1 into each chain back across, sl st 1
back into the stitch you started out from

INSTRUCTIONS

Legs

For the first leg of the doll, form a double loop and insert
hook, then work in tubular rounds as follows:
RND 1: ch 1, sc 10.
RND 2: sc 2 in each stitch around (20 stitches).
RND 3 to RND 25: sc 1 into each stitch around. Sl st 1 to
close round, cut yarn and fasten off.
For the second leg of the doll, follow the same instructions
given for the first but do not cut yarn after round 25, so
that you have one loop left on your hook.

BODY TUBE

Stuff both legs with fiber-fill or toy stuffing, then holding the top edges of the second leg together as shown, ch 2 (replaces first stitch),

and follow the instructions given for the cute doll (Step 3 to Step 8). Proceed with building up the body tube by working in tubular, single crochet rounds until you have 18 rounds. Sl st 1 to close round, cut yarn and fasten off.

ARMS

Form a double loop and insert hook, then work in tubular rounds as follows:

RND 1: ch 1, sc 8.

RND 2: sc 2 in each stitch around (16 stitches).

RND 3 to RND 20: sc 1 into each stitch around. Sl st 1 to close round, cut yarn and fasten off.

Stuff the arm with fiber-fill or toy stuffing, then holding the top edges together as shown in the cute doll instructions, ch 2 (replaces first stitch), *insert hook through two corresponding top edge stitches

(the first stitch and the matching stitch on back) and sc 1*, repeat from * to * until top edge is closed.

Make 2.

HEAD

Form a double loop and insert hook, then work in tubular rounds as follows:

RND 1: ch 1, sc 10.

RND 2: sc 2 in each stitch (20 stitches).

RND 3: *sc 1, sc 2 in the following stitch (1 increase)*; rep from *to* another 9 times (30 stitches).

RND 4: *sc 1 into each of the following 4 stitches, sc 2 into the next stitch (1 increase)* rep from *to* another 5 times

(36 stitches).

RND 5 to RND 13: sc 1 into each stitch around

RND 14: *sc 1 into each of the following 2 stitches, 1 decrease, *; rep from *to* another 7 times (28 stitches).

RND 15: sc 1 into each stitch around

RND 16: decrease 14 (14 stitches)

Sl st 1 to close round. Stuff the head.

Stuff the body tube with fiber-fill or toy stuffing, then close it with a seam, leaving a 14 -stitch opening for attaching the doll's head.

WIG
Step 1, 2, 3

With the bright yellow thread make 7" (18 cm) long decorative fringe embellishments.

Sew the wig onto the head.

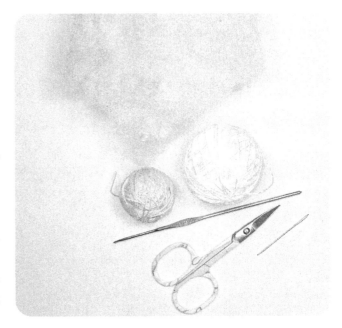

Mini Doll

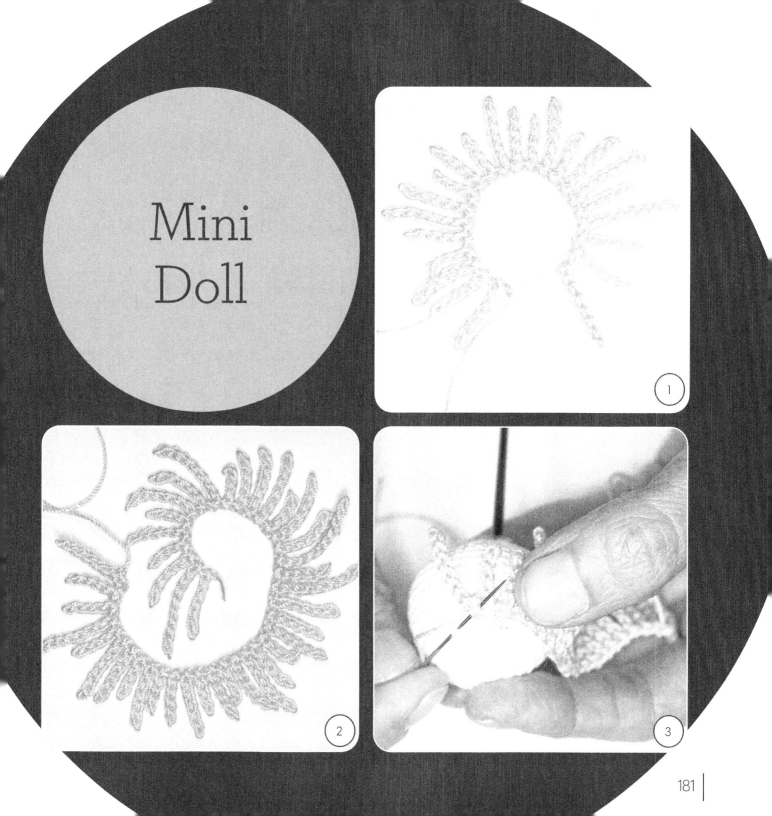

Bonus

As a way to say THANK YOU for starting this journey with me, I have created a bonus project you can find here:

I named it Rainbow Party Crochet Necklace as it's so colorful, it simply makes me smile whenever I wear it. I hope you'll have lots of fun making and wearing it as much as I enjoyed designing it.

Experiment making as many of them as you like in your favorite colors. It makes a perfect gift too!

I can't wait to see your finished pieces inside my Luisa De Santi Crochet Academy! You can access here:

www.facebook.com/groups/luisadesanticrochetacademy

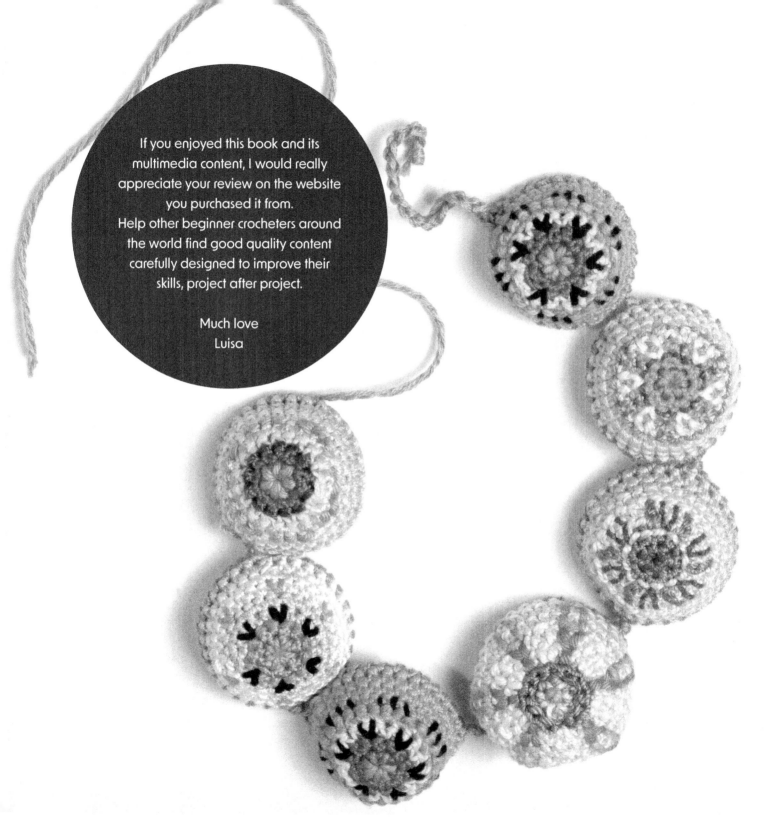

If you enjoyed this book and its
multimedia content, I would really
appreciate your review on the website
you purchased it from.
Help other beginner crocheters around
the world find good quality content
carefully designed to improve their
skills, project after project.

Much love
Luisa